Clinician's Manual on
Treatment of Pediatric Migraine

Clinician's Manual on Treatment of Pediatric Migraine

Donald W. Lewis, MD, FAAP, FAAN
Professor and Chairman
Department of Pediatrics
Children's Hospital of The King's Daughters
Eastern Virginia Medical School
601 Children's Lane
Norfolk, VA. 23507

Disclosures:
The author acknowledges research grant support from:
Abbott Laboratories;
Almirral;
American Home Products;
AstraZeneca;
Boeringer Ingelheim;
GlaxoSmithKline;
Merck;
Ortho McNeil Neurologics

To Penny

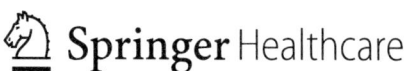

Published by Springer Healthcare Ltd, 236 Gray's Inn Road, London, WC1X 8HL, UK.

www.springerhealthcare.com

©2010 Springer Healthcare, a part of Springer Science+Business Media.

British Library Cataloguing-in-Publication Data.

A catalogue record for this book is available from the British Library.

ISBN 978-1-907673-12-2

Project editor: Tamsin Curtis
Designer: Joe Harvey
Artworker: Sissan Mollerfors
Production: Marina Maher

Contents

Author biography

Dr Lewis, MD, FAAP, FAAN, is a pediatric neurologist at the Children's Hospital of The King's Daughters and Eastern Virginia Medical School in Norfolk, Virginia where he currently serves as Professor and Chairman of the Department of Pediatrics. He has participated in the design and implementation of over 20 clinical trials for migraine in children and authored the American of Academy of Neurology Practice Parameters for the evaluation of the child with recurrent headache and for the pharmacological management of migraine in children and adolescents. He is active in the American Academy of Pediatrics (AAP), serving on the Section of Neurology Board and relishes the opportunity speaking annually at the AAP National Conference Exhibition on the topic of headache. He is fundamentally a clinician-educator and is happiest in the clinic with a medical student on one hip and a resident on the other. His interest in headache began about 25 years ago and has been supported and encouraged by the incomparable, and ever young, Dr David Rothner from the Cleveland Clinic.

Abbreviations

5-HT	5-hydroxytrytamine
AAN	American Academy of Neurology
BM	basilar-type migraine
CDH	chronic daily headache
CGRP	calcitonin gene-related peptide
CoQ10	coenzyme Q10
CSD	cortical spreading depression
CT	computerized tomography
CVS	cyclic (or cyclical) vomiting syndrome
DHE	dihydroergotamine
ECG	electrocardiogram
ED	emergency department
EEG	electroencephalogram
FHM	familial hemiplegic migraine
GI	gastrointestinal
ICHD	International Classification of Headache Disorders
IHS	International Headache Society
IV	intravenous
LA	long acting
MRA	magnetic resonance angiogram
MRI	magnetic resonance imaging
MRV	magnetic resonance venography
NSAIDs	non-steroidal anti-inflammatory drugs
OM	ophthalmoplegic migraine
OTC	over-the-counter
PedMIDAS	Pediatric Migraine Disability Assessment Score
SSRI	selective serotonin reuptake inhibitors
TTH	tension-type headache

Introduction

Migraine is chronic, progressive, debilitating disorder impacting the lives of millions of individuals. The origins of the disability can be traced into childhood and adolescence for the majority adult migraine sufferers [1]. Accurate diagnosis, patient education and aggressive treatment interventions during childhood and adolescence are essential to prevent decades of suffering and diminished quality of life that are directly attributable to migraine. Adequately addressing migraine during adolescence has as much importance on the patient's overall well being as providing immunizations and weight management.

The first step is to make the correct diagnosis. Headache is a very common chief complaint in children and the source of a great deal of angst among both practitioners and parents. Every pediatrician's worst nightmare is missing a brain tumor in a child with headache. Every parent's fear, often unspoken, is that their child's headaches are being caused by a tumor and, as a consequence, many parents demand unnecessary neuro-imaging. Recognizing migraine from the myriad of other types of headaches which present to the office, clinic, or emergency department (ED) requires a straightforward, efficient and systematic process. In addition, knowing when, and when not, it is necessary to perform scans or laboratory tests is essential.

While headaches in children are most often caused by *primary* entities such as migraine or tension-type headache (TTH), the pain may result from *secondary* causes such as brain tumors, idiopathic intracranial hypertension, chronic meningitis, hydrocephalus, paranasal sinus disease, or acute febrile illnesses such as influenza. To determine the cause of a child's headache, the headache evaluation begins with a thorough medical history, followed by methodical physical examination with measurement of vital signs, and with complete neurologic examination. The diagnosis of primary headache disorders such as migraine and TTH rests principally on clinical criteria as set forth by the International Headache Society (IHS) available on line at www.i-h-s.org [2]. Clues to the presence and identification of secondary causes of headache, and thereby the necessity of neuro-imaging, are uncovered through this systematic process of history and physical. The performance of ancillary diagnostic testing rests upon information or concerns revealed during fundamental process.

Diagnosing migraine in young children, or in children with disabilities, can be a particular challenge. The clinical manifestations of migraine vary widely through childhood because the disorder may be expressed incompletely and variably. Mimickers of migraine also emerge during childhood to confuse and complicate the diagnostic landscape. Entities such as epileptic syndromes, congenital malformations, vascular disorders, mitochondrial encephalomyopathies, and metabolic disorders may present with episodic symptoms, including headache. In addition, the medical history can be influenced by the child's ability to articulate the symptoms, coupled with parental interpretation, distortion and editorial. Furthermore, the children are often brought for medical evaluation at the *onset* of transient neurological, autonomic, gastrointestinal (GI), or visual symptoms, before the characteristic recurrent pattern is established, and, curiously, headache may <u>not</u> be the primary symptom. The key aspect to recognizing the spectrum of migraine in children is to appreciate the migraine is an episodic disorder, separated by symptom-free intervals.

The purpose of this manual is to review the epidemiology, classification, pathophysiology, clinical manifestations, and management options for migraine in children and adolescents with an emphasis on those entities peculiar to young children. The **goal** of this manual is to provide a practical toolbox for primary care physicians as they care for children and teenagers with migraine. In the following sections, I hope to provide the reader with the skills to make the right diagnosis and then to fill the toolbox with the various treatment options for the acute treatment and for prevention of migraine in children and adolescents. Except where stated, most of the pharmacological comments will all be off-label.

Chapter 1

Evaluation of the child with headache

The chief complaint of headache in a child or adolescent can be daunting for the busy primary care provider. Having a practical and rational approach to the evaluation of headache in children can make the experience more efficient and effective.

It is important to keep in mind that when parents bring their child to the primary care provider with "headache," there are three questions that they want answered.

1. What is causing the pain?

2. How do we ease the pain?

3. Is there a life-threatening cause, specifically, is there a brain tumor?

Knowing that these are the parent's primary concerns allows us to anticipate and to appreciate their perspective and to set the stage for a successful therapeutic relationship. The third question is foremost in the minds of the parent, the child, and the doctor, so the initial step in the evaluation is to reassure ourselves that there is no underlying life-threatening cause. Once we have satisfactorily reassured ourselves, then we can confidently reassure the family.

To reassure ourselves, we must approach the complaint of headache with the standard medical toolbox of history, physical and neurological examination, followed by appropriate use of ancillary testing. These steps will yield the cause of the headache in the overwhelming majority of children. Once the headache diagnosis is determined, the most appropriate treatment regimen can be formulated from the variety of treatment options discussed in the following sections.

The headache history

The headache database (Figure 1) provides a straightforward series of questions that will help elicit the pertinent features of the headache to help establish a differential diagnosis [3].

Headache database

The basic headache questions

1. What is the pattern of your headache? (explain the different patterns using Figure 2):
   - sudden first headache;
   - episodes of headache;
   - every day headache;
   - gradually worsening; or
   - a mixture (more than one type of headache).

2. How and when did your headache(s) begin?

3. How often do your headaches occur and how long do they last?

4. What makes the headache better or worse?

5. Do any activities, medications, or foods tend to cause or aggravate your headaches?

6. Do the headaches occur under any special circumstances or at any particular time?

The basic medical questions

7. Do you have any other medical problems (high blood pressure, diabetes, epilepsy, neurofibromatosis, tuberous sclerosis)?

8. Are you taking or are you being treated with any medications (for the headache or other purposes)?

The worrisome headache questions; red flag questions

9. Was there any head injury associated with onset of the headaches?

10. Have you ever had seizures or convulsions?

11. Over the past weeks or months have there been any changes in walking, balance, vision, handedness, behavior, speech, or school performance?

12. Have there been any episodes where the headache occurred in the middle of the night or first thing upon awakening? Any vomiting at night or in the morning?

The migraine questions

13. Are there warning signs or can you tell that a headache is coming?

14. Where is the pain located (please point)
   - front;
   - eyes or behind the eyes;
   - side or sides;
   - top;
   - (back) occiput;
   - neck;
   - other?

15. What is the quality of the pain:
   - pounding;
   - squeezing;
   - stabbing; or
   - other?

16. How long do the headaches last?

17. Are there any other symptoms that accompany your headache: nausea, vomiting, dizziness, numbness, lightheadedness, weakness, or other?

Figure 1 Headache database (continues opposite).

Headache database (continued)

18. What do you do when you get a headache or do you have to stop your activities when you get a headache?

19. Does your scalp or face get sensitive to touch during or after a headache (allodynia)?

20. Does anyone in your family suffer from headaches?

Patient's or family's mindset or level of anxiety

21. What do you think might be causing your headache?

Figure 1 Headache database (continued). Adapted from Rothner AD. Semin Pediatr Neurol 1995; 2:109-118.

The questions are organized into five groups.

1. The basic headache questions which establishes the differential diagnosis.

2. The basic medical questions to determine if there are any underlying medical problems.

3. The "RED FLAG" questions which help determine when to worry and who to scan.

4. The "Is this a migraine?" questions.

5. The "What do you think is causing the pain?" question, which gauges the level of anxiety of the patient and their family.

The basic headache questions

The basic headache questions establish the time course and temporal pattern of the headache which, in turn, establishes the differential diagnosis.

Appreciation of the *temporal pattern* (Figure 2) of the patient's headache symptom complex is the most important questions to clarify. This question helps to identify headaches which are more or less likely to be associated with underlying organic pathology, specifically, the ones that will need neuro-imaging. Typically, children's headaches can be separated into one of five patterns.

1. Acute onset of first episode of headache, without prior headache history.

2. Recurring patterns of headache with symptom free intervals.

3. Chronic progressive patterns of increasing headache.

4. Non-progressive daily or near-daily headache.

5. Mixed pattern of daily headache with superimposed more intense attacks (not depicted).

Each of these temporal patterns suggests its own differential diagnosis with headache patterns 1 and 3 being of most concern, the most likely associated with intracranial problems. For example, pattern 1, the acute onset of first episode of headache without a prior history of headache, could be due to a viral illness with fever and, therefore, self limited, but the explosive onset

Four temporal pattern of headaches in children

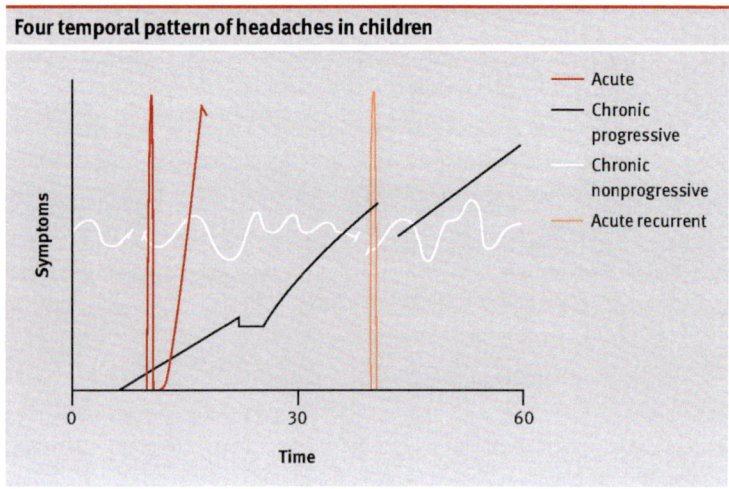

Figure 2 Four temporal pattern of headaches in children. Reproduced with permission from Rothner AD. Semin Pediatr Neurol 1995; 2:109-118.

of headache during straining may suggest a vascular event such as rupture of an aneurysm producing subarachnoid hemorrhage. In the latter instance, an urgent non-contrast head CT scan, followed by spinal fluid analysis is warranted. Contrast that explosive onset of headache to that of a child presenting with a gradually and steadily worsening headache syndrome (pattern 3) accompanied by pain and nausea that awakens her from sleep, the "brain tumor" headache. This child will likely warrant brain Magnetic Resonance Imaging (MRI).

The most commonly encountered form is pattern 2, recurring or episodic headache. This points toward the primary headache disorders such as TTH or migraine. For example, a child with episodes of two-hour length nauseating headaches with periods of interval wellness may be diagnosed by history and physical examination as having migraine, without need for neuro-imaging. Therefore, for patterns 2, 4, and 5, a clinical history and neurological examination alone will generally point toward a specific diagnosis and have the lowest need for neuro-imaging. Whereas, patterns 1 and 3 warrant *consideration* of scans.

"How and when did your headache(s) begin?" Determining how long the headaches have been occurring is quite helpful in assessing the likelihood of an organic cause. The symptoms associated with increased intracranial pressure caused by brain tumors or pseudotumor cerebri (idiopathic intracranial hypertension) will typically evolve over weeks and, very uncommonly, more than three to four months. So, a patient with two years of intermittent headache is highly unlikely to have increased intracranial pressure.

The questions **"How often does the headache occur?"** and **"How long does the headache last?"** helps to identify the characteristic pattern of the individual headache attack. A four-hour attack of pain that occurs once a week would point toward migraine or TTH, whereas very brief, 5–15 min attacks which occur multiple times/day point toward the trigeminal autonomic cephalalgias (ie cluster or paroxysmal hemicrania) or primary stabbing headache.

A standard pain related question is **"What makes the headache better or worse?"** Identification of exacerbating or aggravating phenomena helps both diagnostically and therapeutically. If certain aromas or perfumes or paint fumes trigger off a pounding nauseating headache, the diagnosis is likely migraine and avoidance of the offending agent is a simple intervention.

Medications are frequent and often overlooked causes of headache (Figure 3). Oral contraceptives, non-sedating allergy, or acne medications are frequent causes of headache. Medication overuse as defined by more than five doses of over-the-counter (OTC) agents/week is a common aggravating behavior with Chronic Daily Headache (CDH) and the cycle must be stopped to break the daily pattern.

The food question relates to dietary triggers. Caffeine overuse is an exacerbating phenomena for many teens with migraine or CDH and warrants moderation.

The basic medical questions

This series of questions seeks to identify any underlying medical causes for the pain or any underlying conditions which would predispose to more serious causes for headache (eg neurofibromatosis, epilepsy). The headache database questions also help to identify the co-existence of other symptoms or signs, such as fever, recent trauma, or other medical conditions (eg sickle cell anemia, bleeding diathesis, or autoimmune disorders). The presence of fever with acute headache must raise concerns for viral or bacterial meningitis although in the majority of instances, acute headache with fever is due to self-limited illness such as viral upper respiratory tract infection or pharyngitis.

Drugs that can cause headache

- Oral contraceptives*
- Hormone therapy* (prednisone, dexamethasone, synthroid, anabolic steroids)
- Caffeine (or caffeine withdrawal), ethanol, cocaine
- Non-sedating antihistamines and decongestants
- Ergotamine therapy (DHE), naproxen, ketorolac
- Antihypertensive agents (vasodilators), ACE inhibitors, alpha blockers
- Statins
- Overuse of fat-soluble vitamins, such as vitamin A* and vitamin D
- Sympathomimetics
  – Bronchodilators/β-agonists, methylxanthenes, nalidixic acid, nitrofurantoin, metronidazole
- Atypical antipsychotics, lithium
- Selective serotonin-reuptake inhibitors (SSRI)/SRI
- IV immunoglobulin (IVIG)
- Antibiotics
  – Tetracycline/doxycycline*, amoxicillin, ciprofloxacin, gentamicin

Medications that cause or unmask migraine [4]

- Cyclosporin
- Dipyridamole
- Nitric oxide donors
- Phosphodiesterase inhibitors
- Interferon-b
- Ondansetron
- Tacrolimus
- Fluoxetine
- Sertraline

Medications associated with "overuse headache"

- Aspirin
- Acetaminophen
- Ibuprofen
- Fiorinal/fioricet
- Triptans

Figure 3 Drugs that can cause headache. *Association with idiopathic intracranial hypertension (pseudotumor cerebri); ACE, angiotensin-converting enzyme; DHE, dihydroergotamine; IV, intravenous.

The "Red Flag" questions

Any thorough medical history for headache must include the "Red Flags" which have traditionally been linked to a higher risk of intracranial pathology and must, therefore, trigger consideration of neuro-imaging. This priority list would include:

- patients younger than three years of age;
- early morning pattern or awakening with headache, nausea, or vomiting;
- worsening headache while straining;
- explosive onset (thunderclap headache);
- associated mood, mental status, or school-performance change;
- steadily worsening pattern of headaches (temporal pattern 3); and
- presence of neurocutaneous markers (eg "café au lait" or hypopigmented macules).

These factors should raise concern for ominous problems such as tumors, abscesses, vascular malformations, or bleeds and require prompt consideration for ancillary diagnostic testing (computerized tomography [CT], MRI, Magnetic Resonance Angiogram [MRA], Magnetic Resonance Venography [MRV] and/or electroencephalogram [EEG]).

The "Is this a migraine?" questions

"Are there warning signs or can you tell that a headache is coming?" About a third of migraine sufferers will have an occasional visual or somatosensory (numbness or tingling) aura which lasts 5–30 min and is followed, within a few min, by headache. Stereotypical complex visual auras accompanied by headache and confusion or distortion of consciousness in an elementary age child should also prompt consideration for benign occipital epilepsy. So not all auras point to migraine.

"Where is the pain located and what is the quality of the pain; pounding, squeezing, stabbing, or other?" This question must be asked carefully so as not to "lead the witness." Children will often chose the last of any three choices given to them, so first ask them to describe, demonstrate, gesture, or draw the pain before resorting to a list of choices.

Occipital location may be present in basilar-type migraine (BM) but a steadily worsening, subacute onset of occipital or upper neck pain may indicate the presence of posterior fossa neoplasms such as medulloblastoma or cerebellar astrocytoma.

The question **"Are there any other symptoms that accompany your headache: Nausea, vomiting, dizziness, numbness, weakness, or other?"** seeks to identify the presence of autonomic symptoms but must be carefully explored. Nausea and vomiting are cardinal features of migraine but may also be prominent features of elevated intracranial pressure with brain tumors or idiopathic intracranial hypertension. If the vomiting is occurring while the child is asleep, early in the morning or upon awakening and the child's headaches are gradually and steadily increasing in frequency and severity, then mass lesion must be sought.

Similarly, the complaint of dizziness requires dissection. Does the patient mean lightheadedness, unsteadiness or vertigo? The distinction is important because each suggests differing pathophysiology. Lightheadedness suggests orthostatic hypotension with periodic cerebral hypoperfusion. Unsteadiness or vertigo suggest ataxia or balance disorders pointing toward the cerebellar or vestibular systems, in which case neuro-imaging must be considered. Numbness or weakness likewise must be clarified. Many migraine sufferers will have a peri-oral or hand numbness (chiro-oral) as part of the aura or prelude phase of their attack. The complaint of "weakness" requires exploration as well since many migraine headache patients feel "weak all over," but do not describe a localizable pattern of weakness. A patient who has true weakness such as a hemiparesis with their headache would warrant neuro-imaging in search for intracranial pathology

"What do you do when you get a headache?" or **"Do you have to stop your activities when you get a headache?"** These questions go to the heart of the disability. Do the headaches interfere with activities of daily living? A headache which stops the child in their tracks and forces them to lie down or to ask for medicines is more disabling than a casual mention of headache as the patient passes by on the way out the door to play.

The headache burden or degree of disability imposed by the headache is an essential component of the management decision-making process. Frequent school absences or delayed activities suggest a high headache burden and a more aggressive strategy for prevention. If the disability seems severe, disability rating scales such at the Pediatric Migraine Disability Assessment Score (PedMIDAS) are useful.

An often unrecognized feature, distinctive of migraine, is allodynia, in which the patient will notice that seemingly innocuous sensations are perceived as painful. The question **"Does your scalp or face get sensitive to touch during or after a headache?"** is exploring for the presence of allodynia. Simple acts like brushing hair or applying makeup are quite painful because of the "peripheral sensitization," a phenomenon associated with migraine.

Ask this question **"Does anyone in your family suffer from headaches?"** in an open-ended fashion using the term "headache", not a specific diagnosis such as migraine since, oftentimes, a parent may have migraine but has been mislabeled as sinus or stress headache. Although family history is not one of the diagnostic criteria for migraine, it is, nonetheless, a useful clue to determining if the patient has migraine. This question should also address any other family history of neurological disorders. Brain tumors have an inherited pattern in conditions such as tuberous sclerosis, neurofibromatosis, and von Hippel-Lindau. Also, certain vascular malformations may have heritable patterns (eg cavernous angioma).

The "What do you think might be causing your headache?" question

The patient's and the family's mindset or level of anxiety can be assessed with the question. This question is often the most important one to ask and addresses the inner fears of the patient and their family. The majority of families who present to the office for evaluation of their child's headache are fearful of brain tumors. Recognizing this fact can be extremely useful in establishing confidence and trust. If you are comfortable that the physical and neurological examinations are normal, you can confidently tell the family that there are no signs of brain tumors or anything "bad". Confident reassurance is one of the most potent therapeutic interventions. Conversely, if you have not reassured yourself as to the diagnosis, then further testing or referral may be needed.

Physical and neurological examination

After detailed history, a general physical examination is performed and must include vital signs with blood pressure and temperature looking for signs of hypertension or infection. Also, head circumference must be measured, even in the older children, because slowly progressive increases in intracranial pressure will cause macrocrania. Careful palpation of the head and neck for sinus, jaw, ocular, or TMJ tenderness, thyromegaly, or nuchal rigidity should be performed. Identification of trigger points or areas of maximum tenderness helps to determine the nature of the pain. The skin must also be examined for signs of neurocutaneous syndrome, particularly neurofibromatosis and tuberous sclerosis, which, as stated earlier, are highly associated with intracranial neoplasms.

Following the general physical exam, a detailed neurological examination is essential. This statement is supported by the fact that of the two-thirds of children with brain tumors who present with headache, over 98% will have objective neurological findings. Since reassuring ourselves is fundamental to reassuring our patients, the neurological examination is paramount to providing that essential reassurance.

In the neurological examination, the physician is looking for signs of increased intracranial pressure, integrity of the brain stem, asymmetry of motor or sensory systems, coordination problems, and gait problems. It is important to think about the neurological exam in an anatomical manner so that all of the key regions of the brain are evaluated. For example, the mental status exam assesses the cerebral cortex, cranial nerve exam checks the brain stem function and integrity, motor and sensory systems evaluate the descending and ascending pathways, coordination looks at the cerebellar and vestibular pathways, gait observation puts multiple systems through a dynamic challenge. **The key features include altered mental status, abnormal eye movements, optic disc distortion, motor or sensory asymmetry, coordination disturbances, or abnormal deep tendon reflexes [5].**

The part of the exam that takes practice to master is the fundoscopic exam to assess for papilledema, a sign of increased intracranial pressure. Visualizing the optic discs in young children is often quite a challenge (Figure 4). The key to seeing the optic disc is to have the patient focus their eyes on a far-point, a picture or object directly in front of them. The room should be dimmed, but not dark. The ophthalmoscope is then brought in from the side at about a 30 degree angle to the patient using the examiners right eye to examine the patients right eye (and vice versa) so as not to obstruct the patients focus on the object. This technique allows the physician the best chance to clearly see the optic fundus. Even with practice the fundus cannot always be visualized in the office setting. If there is true concern for increased intracranial pressure as a possible cause of the patient's headaches then a dilated ophthalmoscopic exam may be required.

Visualizing the optic discs in children

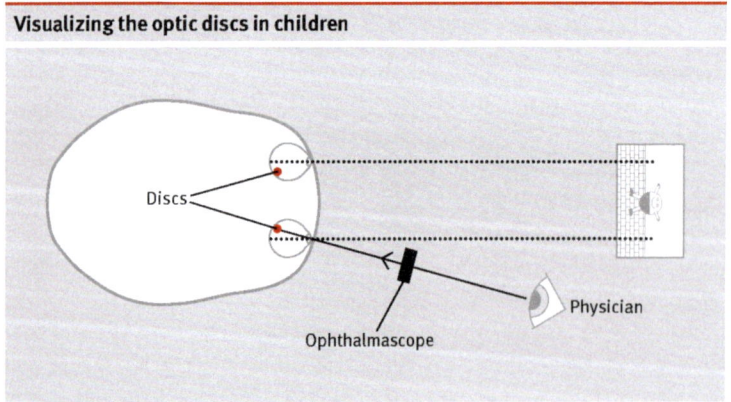

Figure 4 Visualizing the optic discs in children.

Ancillary diagnostic testing: When to worry? When to scan?

Once a detailed history and neurological examination are completed, the appropriate diagnosis can be made in the overwhelming majority of childhood headaches. The next step is to decide if further ancillary diagnostic studies such as laboratory testing, EEG, and neuro-imaging are warranted. The role for such testing for children or adolescents with recurring patterns of headache has been extensively reviewed in the American Academy of Neurology (AAN) Practice Parameter [6] and is available online at www.aan.org.

Routine laboratory testing, while easy to accomplish and relatively inexpensive, has not been found to be beneficial in the diagnosis or evaluation of headaches in children and adolescents. One study of 104 children with headache found that laboratory studies including complete blood count, electrolyte levels, liver function profiles and urinalysis were "uniformly unrevealing" [6]. Given the limited published literature looking at the role of laboratory testing in the evaluation of headaches in children and adolescents the AAN Practice Parameter stated that there is *inadequate documentation* to support any recommendation of routine laboratory studies or performance of lumbar puncture. The practice parameters did not, however, address patients with headache associated with fever or other signs of infection. In this instance, the clinician's best judgment must take precedence.

The AAN Practice Parameter also stated that **routine EEG** *was not recommended* as part of the headache evaluation. Eight studies have assessed the utility of EEG in children with recurrent headaches. The data showed that EEG was not necessary for distinguishing a diagnosis of primary headache disorder in children from secondary headache due to structural disease involving the head and neck, or those due to a psychogenic etiology because the EEG was either normal or demonstrates non-specific abnormalities in the majority of patients [7–15]. Interestingly, even when the EEG was abnormal, it did not provide diagnostic information concerning the etiology of the headache. In addition, EEG is unlikely to distinguish migraine from other types of headaches. Furthermore, children who had paroxysmal EEG's (ie epileptic features) were found to have a negligible risk for future seizures. In fact, none of the patients, whether their EEGs were normal or paroxysmal, subsequently developed seizures. This led to the recommendation from the AAN that "EEG is not warranted in the evaluation of headaches in children or adolescents."

The AAN Practice Parameter from 1994 addressed the utility of neuro-imaging in the evaluation of headache in adults with normal neurologic examinations [16]. The recommendations concluded that **"routine neuro-imaging was unwarranted in patients with recurrent headaches who did not have a recent change in headache pattern, history of seizures, and no focal neurological signs or symptoms."**

Seven pediatric studies addressed the role and rationale for neuro-imaging in children with recurrent headache. One study focused on clinical subsets, migraine and CDH; the remainder included mixed headache subtypes. Based upon these studies, the AAN Practice Parameter explored the role and indications for neuro-imaging for children with recurrent headaches [17–23]. CT scans, MRIs, or both were performed on over 600 children and abnormalities were identified in 16% of the children. However, 82% of these abnormalities were considered to be incidental, non-surgical lesions, or ones that did not require specific medical management. The abnormalities included Chiari malformation, arachnoid cyst without mass effect, paranasal sinus disease, occult vascular malformations, pineal cyst, plus a variety of incidental structural abnormalities such as cavum septi, ventricular asymmetry, and hyperintense lesions.

The most important fact disclosed was that all 18 children who had lesions noted on CT or MRI that were deemed surgically treatable had clear abnormalities such as papilledema, abnormal eye movements, including nystagmus, and motor or gait dysfunction present on neurological examination.

The AAN Practice Parameter made the following recommendations regarding the role of neuro-imaging in the evaluation of children with recurrent headaches.

- Obtaining a neuro-imaging study on a routine basis is not indicated in children with recurrent headaches and normal neurological examinations. Neuro-imaging, however, should be considered in children with an abnormal neurological examination including, but not limited to, focal findings, signs of increased intracranial pressure, significant alteration of consciousness.
- Neuro-imaging should be considered in children in whom there are historical features to suggest the following:
  - a recent onset of severe headache;
  - change in the type of headache;
  - neurological dysfunction; or
  - concerning associated symptoms that accompany the headache.
- Consider neuro-imaging in children who present with headaches and have a co-existence of seizures.

In summary, the evaluation of a child with headache begins with a thorough medical history, followed by methodical physical examination with measurement of vital signs, and with complete neurological examination. Whether or not further testing, including neuro-imaging are needed, rests with this fundamental process.

Once the diagnosis of migraine is established, the spectrum of treatment options can be considered.

Chapter 2

Pediatric migraine

Epidemiology

Headaches are very common during childhood. In Bille's 1962 landmark epidemiological survey of 6000 school children found the prevalence of any headache ranged from 37–51% in seven-year old children and gradually rose to 57–82% by adolescence. Frequent or recurring patterns of headache, of which migraine represents a significant subset, occurred in 2.5% of seven-year olds and up to 15% of 15-year olds [24].

Subsequent epidemiological studies have found that the prevalence of migraine headache steadily increases through childhood, peaking in adolescence. The prevalence rises from 3% in the pre-school ages to 4–11% by elementary school ages, then up to 8–23% during the high school years. Before puberty, boys have more headaches than girls, but following puberty, migraine headaches occur more frequently in girls [25–27].

The incidence (new onset) of migraine peaks earlier in boys than in girls [28]. The mean age of onset of migraine is seven years for boys and 11 years for girls; the gender ratio also shifts during the adolescent years (Figure 5). The incidence of migraine with aura peaks earlier that the incidence of migraine without aura [27, 29–35].

Pathophysiology

Although the pathophysiology of migraine remains unclear, there is a growing body of basic science evidence to support that statement that migraine is a complex *neuroglial* process. Gone are the simple days when migraine was thought to be caused by twitchy blood vessels that constrict and then dilate, to produce symptoms of aura, followed by head pain.

The prevalence of migraine headache through childhood			
By age:	3–7 years	7–11 years	15 years
Prevalence:	1.2–3.2%	4–11%	8–23%
Gender ratio:	boys>girls	boys=girls	girls>boys

Figure 5 The prevalence of migraine headache through childhood.

Migraine is now known to be an inherited *neuroglial* process mediated by a cascade of inflammatory processes around pial and dural blood vessels with the vascular afferents looping back centrally to activate the trigeminal sensory pathways.

One school of thought attributes the whole phenomena of migraine to a hyperexcitable cerebral cortex. The basis of this hyperexcitability is thought to be disturbance of neuronal ion channels, most likely calcium channels, which leads to a lowered cortical electrical threshold, permitting a variety of external and internal factors to trigger electrical waves of *cortical spreading depression* (CSD). In this theory, CSD is the instigating and initiating phenomena for migraine.

CSD begins with episodes of regional neuronal activation, followed by a slowly propagating wave (~2–6 mm/min) of neuronal excitation followed promptly by a wave of neuronal depolarization. CSD explains the migraine aura but the mechanisms and pathways by which CSD activates the *trigeminovascular system* are unclear. Nonetheless, this theory currently has a great deal of traction in the headache community. The holes in this theory are two-fold; how does CSD trigger the neuro-inflammatory cascade and how do we explain the observation that the majority of migraine sufferers do not experience aura?

Clinically, migraine *aura* represents transient, focal, somatosensory symptoms, such as visual scotoma (eg black dots or expanding, shimmering lights) or visual distortions, dysesthesias, hemiparesis, or aphasia. These symptoms are comfortably explained by regional neuronal depolarization and oligemia associated with CSD.

The other prevailing theory regarding migraine pathophysiology is based upon elegant translational research that has demonstrated a neurally-mediated extravasation of plasma inflammatory elements including calcitonin gene-related peptide (CGRP), substance P, nitric oxide, 5-hydroxytrytamine (5-HT) and histamine around dural and pial vessels. This sterile vascular inflammation activates endothelial cells and platelets which add more ingredients into the inflammatory soup such as amines, arachidonate metabolites, peptides and other ions generating a vicious inflammatory cycle [36]. The meningeal vascular inflammation activates trigeminal sensory nerves which send signals centrally, "turning on" brainstem nuclei.

Activation of these brainstem nuclei, specifically, the trigeminal nucleus, the locus ceruleus and dorsal raphi nuclei, is the source of noradrenergic and serotonergic outflow signals that arc back, through the thalamus and ultimately to the cerebral cortex.

The two mechanisms thought to be responsible for the generation of pain in a migraine are: (1) neurogenic inflammation of the meningeal vessels compounded by (2) sensitization of peripheral and central trigeminal afferents.

Sensitization of the trigeminal afferents explains one of the striking features noted during an attack of migraine in which seemingly innocuous activities, such as coughing, walking up stairs, or bending over, greatly intensify the pain. The premise of "sensitization" is that activation of trigeminal vascular afferents stimulate both peripheral and central circuits to become exceptionally sensitive to mechanical, thermal, and chemical stimuli. These circuits become so hypersensitive that virtually any stimulation is perceived as painful, the concept known as *allodynia*. The diagnostic criteria for migraine acknowledge these phenomena by including the phrase "aggravation by routine activities" as one of the essential features of migraine.

These two theories may not be inconsistent with one another, but if CSD is truly the initiating phenomenon that ultimately leads to pain, we must explain how this can occur in the absence of a perceived aura and how CSD initiates neurovascular inflammation. Therefore, the current views of the pathophysiology of migraine suggest an inherited vulnerability to have a hyperexcitable cerebral cortex in which a variety of stimuli may trigger episodes of CSD explaining the aura of migraine. The pain of migraine is generated by neurogenic vascular inflammation with activation and sensitization of both peripheral and central trigeminal afferent circuitry. Unlocking these mechanisms has, and will continue to open the doors to novel treatment measures, such as the triptans, CGRP antagonists, and future targets, such as connexins (gap junction blockers) and glutamate (kainite) receptors.

Classification of pediatric migraine

The International Classification of Headache Disorders (ICHD-2) for migraine is shown in Figure 6 and is available on line at www.i-h-s.org.

There are three principal groups:

1. Migraine without aura.

2. Migraine with aura.

3. Childhood periodic syndromes that are commonly precursors of migraine. Notably absent in the 2004 classification system are several clinical entities peculiar to childhood such as *"Alice in Wonderland"* syndrome, benign paroxysmal torticollis, confusional migraine, and ophthalmoplegic migraine (OM), which will be discussed in the following sections for completeness. Two complications of migraine, status migraine (Chapter 4) and chronic migraine (chapter 5) will be discussed individually later in the book.

Retinal (ophthalmic) migraine, uncommon in childhood, is characterized by fully reversible attacks of monocular positive and/or negative visual phenomena (eg scintillations, scotomata or blindness) confirmed by examination during an attack or by the patient's drawing of a monocular field defect during an attack. The visual symptoms/signs are usually, but not invariably, followed by migraine headache.

International classification of headache disorders: migraine classification

- Migraine without aura
- Migraine with aura
  - Typical aura with migraine headache
  - Typical aura with non-migraine headache
  - Typi al aura without headache
  - Familial hemiplegic migraine
  - Sporadic hemiplegic migraine
  - Basilar-type migraine
- Childhood periodic syndromes that are commonly precursors of migraine
  - Cyclical vomiting
  - Abdominal migraine
  - Benign paroxysmal vertigo of childhood
- Retinal migraine
- Complications of migraine
  - Chronic migraine
  - Status migraine
  - Persistent aura without infarction
  - Migrainous infarction
- Probable migraine

Figure 6 International classification of headache disorders: migraine classification.

Diagnostic criteria for pediatric migraine *without* aura

A. At least 5 attacks fulfilling criteria B–D (below)

B. Headache attacks lasting 1–72 hours

C. Headache has at least two of the following characteristics:
1. Unilateral location, may be bilateral, frontotemporal (not occipital)
2. Pulsing quality
3. Moderate or severe pain intensity
4. Aggravation by or causing avoidance of routine physical activity (eg walking or climbing stairs)

D. During the headache, at least one of the following:
1. Nausea and/or vomiting
2. Photophobia and phonophobia, which may be inferred from their behavior

E. Not attributed to another disorder

Figure 7 Diagnostic criteria for pediatric migraine *without* aura.

Migraine *without* aura

This is the most frequent form of migraine in children and adolescents (60–85%). The diagnostic criteria are shown in Figure 7 and include three modifications to increase sensitivity of diagnosis for children: brief duration (1–72 hours), bilateral/bifrontal location (for patients age <15 years), and the *inference* of photophobia and phonophobia by the child's behavioral response (ie seeking a dark room, turning down volume on TV), rather than verbal report.

The key feature of migraine without aura in children is episodes of intense, disabling headache, separated by symptom-free intervals. The criteria require at least five separate attacks, lasting 1–72 hours and permit attacks to be briefer than in adults, whose migraines typically last 4–72 hours. The location of the pain may be unilateral or, in patients age <15 years, bilateral (bifrontal, bi-temporal) location. The quality of pain is typically pulsing or throbbing, a symptom that may require clarification in young children. By definition, the severity of the pain is moderate to intense and is aggravated by routine physical activity such as walking or climbing stairs. The accompanying associated autonomic features, nausea, vomiting, photophobia, and phonophobia, may be just as disabling as the pain. The IHS criteria wisely also states that the headache must "*not* attributed to another disorder" implying that the prudent physician will carefully consider other possible causes for the recurrent headaches.

Migraine *with* aura

The group of disorders within the spectrum of migraine *with aura* reflects the concept that the focal neurological symptoms such as visual disruptions, hemiparesis, and aphasia are manifestations of regional neuronal depolarization and oligemia caused by CSD. Clinical entities of childhood with focal neurological symptoms, previously termed *"migraine variants"* such as hemiplegic and basilar-type, now are included within this category of migraine with aura or within the group of periodic syndromes (discussed in following sections). Diagnostic criteria for migraine *with* aura are shown in Figure 8.

Approximately 15–30% of children and adolescents with migraine will report visual disturbances, distortions, or obscurations before, or as, the headache begins. The visual symptoms begin gradually and last for several minutes (typical *aura*). The most frequent forms are binocular visual impairment with scotoma (77%), distortion or hallucinations (16%), monocular visual impairment or scotoma (7%) [37]. Formed illusions (eg spots, balloons, colors, rainbows) or other bizarre visual distortions such as macropsia or metamorphopsia, the *"Alice in Wonderland"* syndrome are infrequently reported.

Diagnostic criteria for migraine *with* aura

A. Headache attacks fulfilling criteria for migraine without aura and two attacks fulfilling B–D

B. Aura consisting of fully reversible motor weakness and at least one of the following:
    1. Fully reversible visual symptoms including positive features (eg flickering lights, spots or lines) and/or negative features (eg loss of vision)
    2. Fully reversible sensory symptoms including positive features (eg pins and needles)
    3. Fully reversible dysphasic speech disturbance

C. At least two of the following:
    1. At least one aura symptom develops gradually over ≥5 min
    2. Each aura symptoms lasts >5 and ≤60 min

D. Headache fulfilling criteria migraine without aura begins during the aura or follows aura within 60 min

---

Figure 8 Diagnostic criteria for migraine *with* aura.

If the patient reports the sudden onset of unusual images and complicated visual perceptions, it is prudent to exclude a form of childhood epilepsy known as benign occipital epilepsy [38]. Transient visual obscurations may also be described with idiopathic intracranial hypertension. Therefore, not all visual symptoms with headache are due to migraine with aura.

Basilar-type migraine

Basilar-type migraine (BM) represents 3–19% of childhood migraine and has a mean age an onset of seven years. BM attacks are characterized by episodes of dizziness, vertigo, visual disturbances, ataxia, or diplopia as the aura, followed by the headache phase. The pain of BM may be occipital in location, unlike the usual frontal or bi-temporal pain of typical migraine. The diagnostic criterion requires two or more symptoms and emphasizes *bulbar* and *bilateral* sensorimotor features (Figure 9). Familiar forms of BM linked to the same genes as familial hemiplegic migraine (FHM), types 1 and 2, have recently been reported [39].

Familial hemiplegic migraine

No form of migraine has yielded more information about the underlying molecular genetics of migraine than FHM. FHM, type 1, is an uncommon, autosomal dominant form of migraine *with* aura caused by missense mutation in calcium channel gene (CACNA1A) linked to chromosome 19p13. Clinically, FHM is a migraine headache heralded by an aura which has stroke-like qualities producing some degree of hemiparesis (Figure 10). The transient episodes of focal neurological deficits precede the headache phase by 30–60 min, but, occasionally, extend hours to even days after the headache itself. The location

Diagnostic criteria for basilar-type migraine

A. Fulfills criteria for migraine with aura

B. Accompanied by 2 or more of the following types of symptoms:
   1. Dysarthria
   2. Vertigo
   3. Tinnitus
   4. Hypacusia
   5. Diplopia
   6. Visual phenomena in both the temporal and nasal fields of both of the eyes
   7. Ataxia
   8. Decreased level of consciousness
   9. Decreased hearing
   10. Double vision
   11. Simultaneous bilateral paresthesias

C. At least one of the following:
   1. At least one aura symptom develops gradually over >5 min
   2. Aura symptom lasts >5 min and <24 hours
   3. Headache that fulfills criteria for migraine without aura begins during the aura or follows the onset of aura within 60 min

D. At least one **first-degree or second-degree relative** has had an attack

E. At least one of the following:
   1. History and physical and neurologic examinations not suggesting any organic disorder
   2. History or physical or neurologic examinations suggesting such disorder, but is ruled out by appropriate investigations

Figure 9 Diagnostic criteria for basilar-type migraine.

Diagnostic criteria for familial hemiplegic migraine

A. At least 2 attacks fulfilling criteria B and C

B. Aura consisting of fully reversible motor weakness and at least one of the following:
   1. fully reversible visual symptoms including positive features (eg flickering lights, spots or lines) and/or negative features (ie loss of vision)
   2. fully reversible sensory symptoms including positive features (ie pins and needles) and/or negative features (ie numbness)
   3. fully reversible dysphasic speech disturbance

C. At least two of the following:
   1. at least one aura symptom develops gradually over ≥5 min and/or different aura symptoms occur in succession over ≥5 min
   2. each aura symptom lasts ≥5 min and <24 hours
   3. headache fulfilling criteria B–D for 1.1 migraine without aura begins during the aura or follows onset of aura within 60 min

D. At least one first- or second-degree relative has had attacks fulfilling these criteria

Figure 10 Diagnostic criteria for familial hemiplegic migraine.

of headache is often, but not invariably, contralateral to the focal deficits. Genetic testing is commercially available for FHM type 1.

Many children and adolescents will report transient somatosensory symptoms heralding a migraine attack with focal paresthesias around the mouth and hand (eg chiro-oral aura) without weakness; this does not fulfill the criteria for hemiplegic migraine.

FHM types 2 and 3 are clinically quite similar but have distinctly different molecular mechanisms. FHM type 2 due to point mutation of alpha-2 subunit of the sodium-potassium pump (ATP1A2) gene on chromosome 1q21-23, and type 3 due to sodium channel gene mutation (SCN1A) [40,41].

Sporadic hemiplegic migraine

Sporadic hemiplegic migraine includes those patients who present with the abrupt onset of focal neurological signs or repetitive episodes of focal neurological symptoms *without* family history.

Periodic syndromes of childhood that represent precursors of migraine

Three childhood conditions are included in the category of periodic syndromes; benign paroxysmal vertigo, cyclic (or cyclical) vomiting syndrome (CVS), and abdominal migraine. A fourth, benign paroxysmal torticollis, will be discussed in this section since recent molecular genetic information has demonstrated linkage to migraine. The term *"migraine variants"* was formally applied to this grouping of migraine precursors and some of the forms of migraine with aura, but, today, they are more appropriately categorized according to IHS criterion [42].

Benign Paroxysmal Vertigo occurs in young children with abrupt onset of brief episodes of unsteadiness or ataxia. The child may appear startled or frightened by the sudden loss of balance. Witnesses may report nystagmus or pallor. Verbal children may describe dizziness and nausea. The spells may occur in clusters that typically resolve with sleep. In series of patients available for long-term follow-up, many evolve to basilar-type migraine. The diagnosis of benign paroxysmal vertigo based on a characteristic clinical history, but caution must be exercised to exclude seizure disorders (eg benign occipital epilepsy), otological pathology, posterior fossa lesions, cervical spine abnormalities, familial paroxysmal ataxia, or metabolic disorders.

CVS is characterized by recurrent attacks, usually stereotypical in the individual patient, of vomiting and intense nausea. Attacks are associated with pallor and lethargy. There is complete resolution of symptoms between attacks (Figure 11). Caution must be exercised before making this diagnosis

Diagnostic criteria for cyclic vomiting syndrome

A. At least 5 attacks fulfilling criteria B and C

B. Episodic attacks, stereotypical in the individual patient, of intense nausea and vomiting lasting 1–5 days

C. Vomiting during attacks occurs at least 5 times/hour for at least 1 hour

D. Symptom-free between attacks

E. Not attributed to another disorder. History and physical examination do not show signs of gastrointestinal disease

Figure 11 Diagnostic criteria for cyclic vomiting syndrome.

since episodic vomiting may be seen with a variety of GI, neurological, and metabolic disorders. Once other explanations have been excluded, a significant subset of children with stereotyped episodes of vomiting will have a migrainous basis for their symptoms and represent CVS.

The vomiting episodes occur on regular, often predictable, basis every 2–4 weeks, lasting 1–2 days, and generally begin in the early morning hours. The age of onset is about five years of age and boys and girls are equally affected. While the disorder begins about age five, there is often a significant delay in establishing the diagnosis and most CVS patients are diagnosed at about eight years of age. The majority of children with CVS outgrow their symptoms by age ten. However a significant proportion of patients will have symptoms through adolescence and even as young adults. There is a growing literature about adult CVS.

After a complete diagnostic investigation has excluded other causes of the cyclic vomiting pattern, a comprehensive treatment plan including both acute and prophylactic measures may be instituted. For **acute treatment** of attacks, aggressive hydration, analgesia, sedation, and an anti-emetic agent represent the mainstay. Aggressive oral or intravenous (IV) hydration with a glucose containing solution is essential. Anti-emetic choices include:

- ondansetron (0.3–0.4 mg/kg IV or 4–8 mg oral disintegrating tablet);
- promethazine (0.25–0.5 mg/kg/dose);
- metoclopromide (1–2 mg/kg up to 10 mg bid); or
- prochlorperazine (2.5–5 mg bid).

During an attack, sedation with a benzodiazepine (lorazepam 0.05–0.1 mg/kg up to 5 mg) or diphenhydramine (0.25–1 mg/kg) is often necessary. Ibuprofen (7.5–10 mg/kg orally [po]) may be used for pain.

While not approved by the US FDA for this purpose, there is a growing interest in use of triptan agents for acute episodes of CVS. Subcutaneous sumatriptan (~0.07 mg/kg; maximum 6 mg) has a rapid onset and bypasses the GI tract. Intranasal preparations sumatriptan (5 mg) or zolmitriptan (5 mg) may be tolerated in the vomiting child. If injection or intranasal preparations are not feasible, oral disintegrating tablet forms of rizatriptan or zolmitriptan may have benefit. Again, none of the triptans have been subjected to blinded clinical trials for CVS.

Since the episodes are extra-ordinarily disabling for both the child and their family, it is very reasonable to initiate migraine prophylactic agents for children with CVS. Options include:

- cyproheptadine (2–4 mg/day);
- amitriptyline (5–25 mg/day);
- anticonvulsants such as:
  - divalproex sodium ~10–14 mg/kg/day); or
  - topiramate (1–10 mg/kg/day);
- beta-blockers (eg propranolol); or
- calcium channel blockers (eg verapamil).

Abdominal migraine is an idiopathic, recurrent disorder seen mainly in children and characterized by episodes of vague anterior midline or periumbilical abdominal pain lasting 1–72 hours with complete resolution of symptoms between attacks. The pain is of moderate to severe intensity and associated with vasomotor symptoms, nausea and vomiting (Figure 12). Abdominal migraine includes a subset of patients with chronic, recurrent abdominal pain that have features which overlap with those of migraine without aura. Abdominal migraine generally occurs in school-aged children, who report recurrent attacks of midline, or upper abdominal, pain that is dull in nature and generally lasts for hours. About 5–15% of children with idiopathic recurrent abdominal pain will meet the diagnostic criteria for abdominal migraine.

Diagnostic criteria for abdominal migraine

A. At least 5 attacks fulfilling criteria B–D

B. Attacks of abdominal pain lasting 1–72 hours

C. Abdominal pain has all of the following characteristics:
   1. midline location, periumbilical, or poorly localized
   2. dull or "just sore" quality
   3. moderate or severe intensity

D. During abdominal pain, at least 2 of the following:
   1. anorexia
   2. nausea
   3. vomiting
   4. pallor

E. Not attributed to another disorder. History and physical examination do not show signs of gastrointestinal or renal disease or such disease has been ruled out by appropriate investigations

Figure 12 Diagnostic criteria for abdominal migraine.

As with CVS, the key to this entity is to recognize the recurrent pattern of symptoms and to exclude other GI or renal diseases by appropriate investigations. An up to date reference list for CVS and abdominal migraine is available on line at *www.cvsaonline.org*.

An uncommon entity which has historically been included in the spectrum of migraine variants, but omitted from the IHS grouping of periodic syndromes, is *Benign Paroxysmal Torticollis*. This disorder is a uncommon paroxysmal movement disorder (dyskinesia) characterized by attacks of head tilt or head tilt accompanied by vomiting and ataxia that may last hours to days. Other twisting, tortional or dystonic features, including truncal or pelvic posturing, may be seen. Curiosly attacks first manifest during infancy between two and eight months of age.

Paroxysmal torticollis is likely an early onset variant of BM but the differential diagnosis must include gastro-esophogeal reflux (Sandifer syndrome), idiopathic torsional dystonia, complex partial seizure, but particular attention must be paid to the posterior fossa and craniocervical junction where congenital or acquired lesions may produce torticollis. Once the diagnosis is established and the benign nature confirmed, there may be no requirement for treatment beyond reassurance.

Investigators in the UK have found a linkage to the CACNA1-A gene in families with paroxysmal torticollis which may bring this disorder back into the family of periodic syndromes in future revisions of the ICHD classification system [43].

Other unusual forms of migraine in childhood

"Alice in Wonderland" syndrome represents the spectrum of *migraine with aura*, but the visual aura is quite atypical and may include bizarre visual illusions and spatial distortions preceding an otherwise nondescript headache. Affected patients will describe distorted visual perceptions such as micropsia, macropsia, metamorphopsia, teleopsia, or macro/microsomatognopsia. The visual symptoms likely represent CSD and oligemia involving the parieto-occipital region heralding the headache.

Confusional migraine has perceptual and cognitive distortions as its cardinal feature. Affected patients, usually boys, abruptly become agitated, restless, disoriented, and occasionally combative. The confusion phase may last minutes to hours. Later, once consciousness returns to baseline, the patients will describe an inability to communicate, frustration, confusion, loss of orientation to time, and may *not* recall a headache phase at all. Confusional migraine often occurs following seemingly innocuous head injury that occurs in sports (eg soccer, football, skating) and can be included in the spectrum of trauma-triggered migraine. Clearly, any sudden unexplained alteration of consciousness following head injury warrants investigation for intracranial hemorrhage, drug intoxication, metabolic derangements and epilepsy.

Clinically, confusional migraine most likely represents an overlap between hemiplegic migraine and basilar-type migraine. Patients who present with unilateral weakness or language disorders should be classified as hemiplegic migraine and patients with vertiginous or ataxic patterns classified as BM.

Ophthalmoplegic migraine (OM) has been removed from the migraine spectrum into the group of cranial neuralgias as a result of elegant neuro-imaging evidence which demonstrated an underlying demyelinating-remyelinating mechanism. The key clinical feature is *painful ophthalmoparesis.* The pain may be a nondescript ocular or retro-ocular discomfort. Ptosis, limited adduction, and vertical displacement (eg cranial nerve III) are the most common objective findings. The oculomotor symptoms and signs may appear well into the headache phase, rather than heralding the headache, contrary to the sequence of typical migraine. The signs may persist for days or even weeks after the headache has resolved. Since OM is no longer viewed as migraine, eventually, the term "ophthalmoplegic migraine" will likely evolve to ophthalmoplegic *neuralgia* or *neuralgiform disorder.*

The migraine precursors and these unusual forms of migraine with aura are unique to pediatrics and represent a challenging group of disorders characterized by the abrupt onset of focal neurological signs and symptoms (eg hemiparesis, altered consciousness nystagmus, or ophthalmoparesis) followed by headache. Frequently, these ominous neurological signs initially point the clinician in the direction of epileptic, cerebrovascular, traumatic, or metabolic disorders and only after thorough neuro-diagnostic testing does the migraine diagnosis become apparent. Some of these entities occur in infants and young children where history is limited. Only after careful history, physical, and appropriate neuro-diagnostic studies can these diagnoses be comfortably entertained. All of these disorders represent diagnoses of exclusion.

Chapter 3

Management options for pediatric migraine

Once the diagnosis of migraine is established, a balanced, flexible and individually tailored treatment plan can be put in to place. It is important to educate the patient and their family about the diagnosis of migraine and to provide reassurance about the absence of other, life-threatening disorders. Invariably, families have a fear of an underlying malignancy and it is absolutely essential to provide reassurance. Once this point is established, the family will get "on board" with the treatment regimen.

The fundamental goals of long-term migraine treatment have been established:

- reduction of headache frequency, severity, duration, and disability;
- reduction of reliance on poorly tolerated, ineffective, or unwanted acute pharmacotherapies;
- improvement in the quality of life;
- avoidance of acute headache medication escalation;
- education and enablement of patients to manage their disease to enhance personal control of their migraine; and
- reduction of headache-related distress and psychological symptoms [44].

To achieve these goals, the treatment regimen must balance *bio-behavioral strategies and pharmacological measures.*

When developing the individualized treatment plan, the first step is to appreciate the *degree of disability* imposed by the patient's headache. Understanding of the impact of the headache on the quality of life will guide in the decisions regarding the most appropriate therapeutic course [45,46].

Bio-behavioral therapies (non-pharmacologic measures)

Bio-behavioral treatments include: sleep hygiene, exercise, dietary modifications, and the repertoire of psychological interventions including biofeedback, guided imagery, cognitive control, hypnosis, and stress management (Figure 13). The value of these interventions cannot be overstated. *Virtually every migraine sufferer* will benefit from a basic review of these measures, but the patient with more frequent attacks or daily migraine (CDH) who has a greater the degree of disability will have a greater need to comply with these measures.

Good **sleep hygiene** is essential for adolescents with frequent migraine headaches. Chaotic sleep patterns, staying up late on weekends, sleeping in until afternoon on Saturday and Sunday, and then getting up early for school on Monday, sets the stage for Monday morning migraines. Sleep disturbances have been found to occur in 25–40% of children with migraine. Too little sleep (42%), bruxism (29%), co-sleeping (sleeping with parents or other family member) (25%), and snoring (23%) were found among a population of 118 children using the Children's Sleep Habit Questionnaire. When children with migraine were compared with matched controls, statistically

---

Bio-behavioral therapies for pediatric migraine

- Identification of migraine triggers
- Biofeedback
  - Electromyographic biofeedback
  - Electroencephalography biofeedback
  - Thermal hand warming biofeedback
  - Galvanic skin resistance biofeedback
- Relaxation therapy
  - Progressive muscle relaxation
  - Autogenic training
  - Meditation
  - Passive relaxation
  - Self-hypnosis
- Cognitive therapy/Stress management
  - Cognitive control
  - Guided imagery
- Dietary measures
  - Avoidance diets
  - Caffeine moderation
  - Herbs
    - Butterbur root
    - Feverfew (Tanacetum parthenium)
    - Ginkgo
    - Valerian root
  - Minerals
    - Magnesium
  - Vitamins
    - Riboflavin (B2)
- Acupuncture
- Aroma therapy

Figure 13 Bio-behavioral therapies for pediatric migraine.

significant differences were found in sleep duration, daytime sleepiness, night wakening, sleep anxiety, parasomnias, sleep onset delay, bedtime resistance, and sleep-disordered breathing [47]. The authors of this study stated that it is unclear, however, whether sleep disturbances increased the occurrence of migraine, whether frequent and intense migraine lead to sleep disturbances, or whether the two are unrelated. Clearly, further investigation is necessary. Current clinical practice is to recommend good sleep hygiene.

A regular **exercise** program is recommended for adolescents with frequent migraines. A recent study evaluated the effects of exercise and plasma endorphin levels in 40 migraine patients. Beneficial effects were found on all migraine parameters [48].

Some basic dietary recommendations include three square meals per day, including breakfast. Many teens routinely skip breakfast and get headaches in the late morning. This is a simple recommendation, but many busy families find this recommendation onerous. Hydration is often inadequate in children with migraine, so 4–5 extra glasses of water (not soda) per day can solve that problem.

The role of **diet** remains controversial [49]. Somewhere between 7–44% of patients will report that a particular food or drink can precipitate a migraine attack [50,51]. In children, the principal dietary triggers were cheese, chocolate, and citrus fruits. Wholesale dietary elimination of a list of foods is, however, not recommended. Elimination diets are excessive and set the stage for a battleground at home when parents attempt to enforce a restrictive diet upon an unwilling, resistant adolescent. The ensuing family friction may ultimately heightened tensions at home, worsening the headache pattern. A more reasonable approach is to review the list of foods thought to be linked to migraine and encourage the patient to keep a headache diary to see if a temporal relationship exists between ingestion of one or more of those foods and the development of headache. If a link is discovered, common sense dictates avoidance of the offending food substance.

Caffeine warrants special mention. A link between caffeine and migraine has been established [52,53]. Not only does caffeine itself seem to have a negative influence on headache; caffeine may disrupt sleep or aggravate mood, both of which may exacerbate migraine. Furthermore, caffeine withdrawal headache, which begins 1–2 days following cessation of regular caffeine use, can last up to one week [54]. Every effort must be made to moderate caffeine use.

The basic recommendations given to migraine sufferers include regular sleep and exercise, moderation of caffeine intake, and adequate hydration.

Psychological interventions

The role of **psychological interventions** cannot be overstated. Biofeedback, stress management, hypnosis, guided imagery, and cognitive control are underutilized therapeutic interventions which have been subjected to controlled trials and good evidence supports their value [55]. Specific techniques involved is beyond the scope of this monograph and the typical primary care provider will not have the skill set, or time, to provide these services. The most practical approach is to be aware of providers (child psychologists, licensed clinical social workers, counselors) in your geographic region who are trained in these interventions and establish a clinical partnership. Since pain management spans many pediatric disciplines (oncology, rheumatology, sports medicine, gastroenterology, neurology), having individuals in your immediate healthcare network skilled and confident in these techniques is invaluable. One very valuable reference is **Conquering Your Child's Chronic Pain** by Zeltzer and Schlank [56]. This book has helped many families to understand the concepts of chronic pain and value of psychological therapies.

Complementary and alternative therapies

Within Figure 13 are included some of the complementary and alternative treatment therapies (CAM) for pediatric and adult migraine. Few have been subjected to controlled trials in children, but nonetheless have become commonly used and recommended widely on patient-education websites. Many families embrace CAM therapies and are suspicious of traditional medicines.

Both magnesium (~400–800 mg/day) and riboflavin (B2) (~400 mg/day) have demonstrated efficacy in controlled prophylaxis trials and are currently recommended for the prevention of migraine in adults [57]. Data regarding other herbal remedies is limited in children. Butterbur root, for example, was compared to placebo and music therapy, and only music therapy showed superiority compared to placebo during the trial period, but during extended follow up, both music therapy and butterbur showed value [58].

An intriguing study was conducted by Hershey et al to explore the value of coenzyme Q10 (CoQ10) in the management of migraine. The authors measured the levels of CoQ10 in 1550 children and found that 33% had values less than reference range. These patients were supplemented with 1–3 mg/kg/day of CoQ10 and in follow up their headache frequency improved from 19 headaches (+/- 10) to 12 (+/- 11)/month ($p < 0.001$). The authors proposed that CoQ10 deficiency may be a common phenomenon in children with frequent migraine [59]. This clearly warrants further study.

Pharmacological management

The pharmacological management of pediatric migraine has been subjected to thorough review but controlled data is, unfortunately, limited; therefore, most of the below recommendations are all off label [60–64].

Acute treatment

Acute treatments represent the mainstay of migraine management. The patient should be offered several acute treatment options after the initial office visit, so that they may determine what medicines work most effectively for them. Regardless of the acute treatment selected, there are several basic guidelines regarding the use of acute treatments which must be included as part of the patient's educational process. The essential message is *give enough and give it early*!

- Take the medicine as soon as possible when the headache begins; within 20–30 min; it is okay to take the medicine when the headache is still mild.
- Take the appropriate dose; do not "baby" the headache, "nuke" it!
- Have the medicine available and accessible at the location where the patient usually has their headaches (eg school). Complete the school medicine forms with clear guidelines and dosing instructions to the school nurse.
- Avoid analgesic overuse (>3 doses of analgesic/week). Overuse of OTC analgesics (>3–5 times/week) can be a contributing factor to frequent, even daily, headache patterns. When recognized, patients who are overusing analgesics must be educated to discontinue the practice. Retrospective studies have suggested that this recommendation alone can decrease headache frequency [65,66].

For the acute treatment of migraine, the most rigorously studied agents are ibuprofen, acetaminophen, and selected triptans (rizatriptan and almotriptan tablets, sumatriptan and zolmitriptan nasal sprays), all of which have shown safety and efficacy in controlled trials in children and/or adolescents (Figure 14). While the triptans have revolutionized acute migraine treatment for adults, only one, almotriptan, has been approved by the FDA for use in adolescents, even though multiple studies have demonstrated the safety of triptans in children [67,68].

For young children, age <12 years, ibuprofen (7.5–10 mg/kg) and acetaminophen (15 mg/kg) have demonstrated efficacy and safety for the acute treatment of migraine [69,70].

For teenagers, four triptans, two in tablet form and two in the nasal spray form have demonstrated efficacy. The tablet forms of rizatriptan (5 and 10 mg) and almotriptan (6.25, 12.5, and 25 mg) and the nasal spray forms

Options for acute treatment for pediatric migraine

Drug	Trade name	Dosing form
Acetaminophen† (10–15 mg/kg/dose)		80, 160, 325 mg tablets 160 mg/tsp syrup
Ibuprofen† (7.5–10 mg/kg/dose)		100 mg chewable tablets 100 mg/tsp syrup 200, 400, 600, 800 mg tablets
Naproxen sodium (2.5–5 mg/kg/dose)		220 (OTC), 250, 375, 500 mg
5-HT agonists (TRIPTANS)		
Almotriptan*†	AXERT	12.5 mg
Rizatriptan†	MAXALT	5, 10 mg tablets 5, 10 mg disintegrating tablet
Sumatriptan†	IMITREX	25, 50, 100 mg tablets 6 mg subcutaneous injection 5, 20 mg nasal spray†
Sumatriptan/ naproxen combination†	TREXIMET	85 mg sumatriptan/500 mg naproxen
Zolmitriptan†	ZOMIG	2.5, 5 mg tablets 2.5, 5 mg disintegrating tablet 5 mg nasal spray†

Figure 14 Options for acute treatment for pediatric migraine. †Supportive efficacy and safety data in adolescents. *US FDA approved for use in adolescents age 12–17 years; OTC, over-the-counter.

of sumatriptan (5 and 20 mg) and zolmitriptan (5 mg) have demonstrated both safety and efficacy in controlled trials in adolescents, age 12–17 years (Figure 14) [71–76]. Treximet™, a combination agent with sumatriptan (85 mg) plus naproxen (500 mg) has demonstrated safety and efficacy in adults and recent data in adolescents has shown safety and tolerability, but efficacy in adolescents has not yet been demonstrated [77,78]. Almotriptan is the only triptan currently approved by the US FDA for the acute treatment of migraine in adolescents.

The evidence for acute treatments in children and adolescents

Simple analgesics and non-steroidal anti-inflammatory drugs (NSAIDs) are quite effective in children and adolescents. Many families will dismiss the suggestion of simple analgesics because they "already tried that." Oftentimes, however, the family has not used the appropriate dose and, more importantly have not treated within the critical 30 min window of opportunity. Don't jump to the more expensive agents until an adequate trial of ibuprofen has been given.

Ibuprofen

Ibuprofen (7.5–10 mg/kg) has been shown in three double-blind, placebo-controlled trials to be safe and effective in the treatment of childhood migraine. The first study compared ibuprofen (10 mg/kg) to acetaminophen (15 mg/kg) and placebo. Both ibuprofen (68% active vs 37% placebo) and acetaminophen (54% vs 37%) were significantly more effective than placebo in providing pain relief at two hours. Differences between ibuprofen compared to acetaminophen were not statistically significant at two hours. Acetaminophen was considered effective and well tolerated. In the second study, ibuprofen (7.5 mg/kg) was found to reduce headache severity in children ages 6–12 years, but was significant at the two hour primary endpoint, but only in boys. The third study which also included a zolmitriptan arm, showed ibuprofen to be effective (69% vs 28%) [79]. No statistically significant adverse effects of ibuprofen or acetaminophen were reported from these studies [69,70]. Ibuprofen works in two-thirds to three-quarters of patients.

The 2004 AAN Practice Parameter has found that "ibuprofen is *effective* and should be considered for the acute treatment of migraine in children." In addition, the parameter concludes that "acetaminophen is *probably effective* and should be considered for the acute treatment of migraine in children."

Naproxen

Naproxen has not been studied in any controlled fashion for the acute treatment of pediatric migraine but clearly warrants consideration among the therapeutic options. Two advantages to naproxen are its relatively longer duration of action than ibuprofen or acetaminophen and its lower tendency to cause analgesic overuse headache. The dose of naproxen is 5 mg/kg/dose with a maximum dose per day being 15 mg/kg/day; it may be administered two to three times/day in liquid (250 mg/5cc) or tablet form (250, 375, 500 mg).

The triptan agents

The introduction of the 5-hydroxytryptamine (5-HT1) agonists, a class of agents known as the triptans has revolutionized the treatment of migraine attacks in adults. Multiple controlled trials in adolescents have demonstrated the safety of the triptans. Efficacy, however, has only been demonstrated with almotriptan tablets and in the nasal spray forms of sumatriptan and zolmitriptan. Almotriptan is the only triptan approved by the US FDA for use in adolescents 12–17 years whose migraines last more than four hours.

Nonetheless, children and adolescent who have not had sufficient relief from acetaminophen, ibuprofen, or naproxen may be candidates for the triptans. In our practice, the most commonly used triptans are almotriptan tablets (12.5 mg), sumatriptan nasal spray (20 mg) and tablets (25, 50, 100 mg), zolmitriptan nasal spray (5 mg) and oral disintegrating tablets (2.5, 5 mg), and rizatriptan oral disintegrating tablets (5, 10 mg).

Caution should be exercised with the triptan class if there is a history of hypertension, use of monoamine oxidase inhibitors, basilar or hemiplegic migraine, or family history of early coronary artery disease. A clear contraindication would be any past history of ischemic heart disease.

Common side effects include flushing and neck, jaw, and chest tightness. These are unusual side effects for children to experience so it is important to alert the patient and family. The nasal spray preparations also have an issue with bad taste if the medicine drips over the palate. Proper training to demonstrate the administration of the nasal sprays, with avoidance of snorting the spray, can minimize this noxious taste. It is important to aim the spray toward the upper nose and to keep the head upright following administration. The patient is coached to avoid sucking the medicine back into the oropharynx, where it can be tasted. In addition, the disturbance in taste may be mitigated in many patients by the use of flavored lozenges or hard candy (ie butterscotch) after administration of the nasal spray. Some migraine sufferers are willing to tolerate the bad taste given the beneficial effects on their headaches.

Cardiac toxicity has been observed in very rare instances in adolescents with co-morbid hypertension, obesity, and diabetes. If significant cardiovascular risk factors are uncovered, triptans should be used with caution.

Almotriptan

Almotriptan (Axert™) is a novel serotonin 5-$HT_{1B/1D}$ receptor agonist and exerts its actions upon receptors located on the extracerebral and intracranial pial and dural blood vessels which become dilated during a migraine attack and upon trigeminal nerve endings. Activation of these serotoninergic receptors results in vasoconstriction, inhibition of inflammatory neuropeptide release, and reduction of transmission in trigeminal pain pathways, essentially inhibiting the pathophysiologic mechanisms of migraine at several levels [80].

Almotriptan has a half-life of about three hours and is well absorbed after oral dosing with nearly 70% of maximum plasma concentrations being reached in one hour. Food does not alter absorption and, in addition, absorption is not altered during a migraine attack. The bioavailability of almotriptan is the highest among all the triptans. The pharmacokinetic parameters do not differ between adults and adolescents [80]. Two open-label, uncontrolled, trials demonstrated the safety of almotriptan in adolescents. A small study of 15 children, ages 11–17, found "virtually no adverse effects" other than transient neck stiffness and was deemed "effective" in 13/15 patients. The author concluded that almotriptan is "probably safe and effective" in this age range [81].

A second open-label study assessed the long term safety of 12.5 mg oral almotriptan in 420 adolescents, 319 of whom completed the 12 month study. The patients treated over 8000 migraine attacks and reported pain relief of 62% and 69% at 2 and 24 hours with a sustained pain relief rate of 56%, although there was no placebo arm. Absence of pain at 2 hours was observed in 40%. About 73% of the patients required a second 'rescue' dose of 12.5 mg for at least one of their migraine attacks. The authors noted that the most optimal responses were observed among adolescents who took almotriptan when the pain was mild. Over 7% of patients reported side effects including nausea and somnolence. About 2% experience adverse effects prompting them to discontinue use of almotriptan [82].

Almotriptan has recently been approved by the US FDA based on data from a randomized study of 866 adolescents who received 6.25, 12.5, or 25 mg doses versus matched placebo [76]. The results demonstrated headache relief (defined as a two point reduction in pain on a four point scale) at a two hour endpoint in 72%, 73%, and 67% versus 55% for the placebo with statistical significance being reached with the 6.25 and the 12.5 mg doses. Interestingly, the study designers used a bold composite primary endpoint of migraine relief, meaning relief of pain *and* associated symptoms, which failed to reach statistical significance. Nonetheless, the gold standard for migraine trials has been headache relief at two hours, a secondary endpoint in this study which did achieve significance.

The recommended dose of almotriptan in adolescents is 6.25 mg or 12.5 mg at the onset of a migraine attack. If the migraine returns after two hours, a second dose may be administered, but no more than 25 mg should be taken in 24 hours.

Rizatriptan

Rizatriptan (Maxalt™) is available in 5 mg and 10 mg tablets and oral disintegrating tablets. There is excellent data to support the use of rizatriptan in children, as young as six years of age, and adolescents. Investigators in Finland conducted a triple-blind cross-over trial in 96 children (age 6–17 years) and found headache relief in 74% of patients receiving rizatriptan and 36% in those receiving placebo (p<0.001). Their findings held up following multiple attacks [75].

An earlier study of adolescents ages 12–17 years (n=149) in a double-blind, placebo-controlled, parallel-group, single-attack design with 5 mg dosing found pain relief at two hours for the rizatriptan group was 66%, but the response of the placebo group was 57% (p=NS). The response rate was better on weekends. Functional disability was significantly improved with rizatriptan 5 mg (44%) compared with the placebo group (36%). There were no serious adverse events and the most common adverse events reported were fatigue, dizziness, somnolence, dry mouth, and nausea [83].

Sumatriptan

Sumatriptan (Imitrex™) has been the most rigorously studied triptan in adolescents. Available in tablet, nasal spray, and subcutaneous injection form, and the oral tablets and nasal formulations are preferable for use in children.

Oral sumatriptan has been studied in a double-blind, placebo-controlled trial of 25, 50, and 100 mg tablets in 302 adolescents at 35 sites. Response to sumatriptan met statistical significance when compared to placebo at 25, 50, and 100 mg at the 180 and 240 min mark showing 74% pain relief at the four hour mark, however the primary endpoint of the study was at two hours, and statistical significance was *not* reached [84].

Sumatriptan nasal spray has been studied in three controlled trials has demonstrated both efficacy and safety in adolescent migraine. The first study (n=14) found significant headache relief at two hours in 85.7% vs 42.9% in the placebo group (p=0.03). Headache-associated symptoms were also significantly improved in the sumatriptan group; nausea decreased by 36% and phonophobia by 57% [85].

The second study was multicenter, double-blind, placebo-controlled and included 510 adolescents, ages 12–17 years, comparing 5, 10 and 20 mg sumatriptan nasal spray to placebo. The two hour response rate, defined as reduction in headache severity from severe or moderate to mild or no headache, was 66% for the 5 mg dose (p<0.05), 63% for the 20 mg dose (p=0.059), and 53% for placebo. Significant relief was noted at one hour in the 5 mg and 20 mg dosing arms (p<0.05). A pain free state at two hours was achieved to a statistically significant degree with 20 mg nasal spray (p<0.05). Both photophobia and phonophobia were reduced with the 20 mg dose (p<0.05). The only adverse effect was taste disturbance (26%) [71].

The third trial, a double-blind, placebo-controlled, two-way crossover design (n=83), included younger children (ages 8–17 years) with a median age of 12.4 years. Doses of 10 mg nasal spray were provided for children weighing

20–39 kg and 20 mg for children weighing >40 kg. The primary endpoint was headache relief as defined by a two point improvement in headache severity based upon a five point pain scale at two hours. At two hours, the primary endpoint was met in 64% of patients receiving sumatriptan and in 39% of those receiving matching placebo (p=0.003). At one hour, headache relief was found in 51% of children receiving sumatriptan and in 29% receiving placebo (p=0.014). Complete pain relief was experienced by 31% of those treated with sumatriptan and 19% receiving placebo (p=0.14). Secondary endpoints including use of rescue medications and patient preference also "favored" sumatriptan nasal spray. Bad taste was again the most common side effect (29%) [72]. Taste disturbance is the most common problem encountered with sumatriptan nasal spray.

Overall, sumatriptan nasal spray 20 mg provided the most rapid treatment across this adolescent population group. The 2004 AAN Practice Parameter has found that sumatriptan nasal spray "is effective and should be considered for the acute treatment of migraine in adolescents."

One open-label trial of the effectiveness of **subcutaneous sumatriptan** (0.06 mg/kg) showed an overall efficacy of 72% at 30 min and 78% at two hours, with a recurrence rate of 6%. Due to children's tendency to report shorter headache duration, a recurrence rate of 6% would seem appropriate for this study population [86]. The obvious limitation to the use of a subcutaneous preparation is a child's aversion to injections.

Zolmitriptan

Zolmitriptan (Zomig™) was studied in adolescents (n=38) who entered in a one year open label trial. The first two migraine subgroups were treated with 2.5 mg tablets and subsequent attacks with 2.5 or 5 mg tablets at each patient's discretion. The overall headache response at two hours was 80% (88% and 70% with zolmitriptan, 2.5 and 5 mg, respectively) and treatment was well tolerated [87].

A clinical trial of zolmitriptan nasal spray (5 mg) used a novel enrichment design in an attempt to mitigate the high placebo response rate seen in previous adolescent trials. Each study subject initially treated a migraine attack with a placebo nasal spray within 30 min of the onset of their headache (single-blind phase). If a headache response was obtained at 15 min, no further medication was taken. Those patients with ongoing headache of moderate to severe intensity 15 min after the first (placebo) spray then took either active agent or matched placebo (double-blind phase). Zolmitriptan nasal spray demonstrated a headache response rate at one hour post-dose superior to placebo (58.1% vs 43.3%; p<0.02). The onset of action was early as 15 min. The two hour sustained headache response rate for zolmitriptan nasal spray was 53.4% vs 36.2% for placebo (p<0.01). Patients treated with zolmitriptan nasal spray, 51% were able to return to normal activities at one hour versus 37.5% treated with placebo (p<0.03). There were no serious adverse events, no withdrawals due to adverse events and there was a low incidence of adverse events, with unusual taste (dysgeusia) being the most common side effect (6.5%) [88].

Other triptans

Naratriptan, frovatriptan, and eletriptan have not been extensively studied in children and adolescents. Naratriptan and frovatriptan have a long duration of action and have demonstrated value in women with menstrual migraine.

Dihydroergotamine

Intranasal dihydroergotamine (DHE) (Migranal™) has not been formally evaluated in children or adolescents. Nonetheless, patients who respond to IV DHE for status migraine may benefit from its use. Co-administration with anti-emetics may be necessary since DHE can cause intense nausea. IV DHE is discussed in the following section on status migraine. DHE should not be used within 24 hours of a triptan.

Combination agents

Butalbital preparations, once a mainstay of headache treatment, have been supplanted by the current generation of migraine-specific agents. The combination of aspirin and acetaminophen warrants caution because of the aspirin which used very cautiously in children, particularly if the child has had or is having a febrile illness. Use of butalbital preparations should be discouraged. Likewise, isometheptine/dichloralphenzazone/acetaminophen combinations (Midrin™), never studied in adolescents, is less commonly used with the other available agents.

Antiemetics

For many children with migraine, the accompanying symptom of nausea or vomiting can be just as disabling as the pain. Antiemetics, available in suppository, oral, sublingual, or parenteral forms, are extremely useful in children and adolescents with acute migraine that is accompanied by disabling nausea or vomiting. Commonly used agents are shown in Figure 15.

Commonly used anti-emetics*

Drug	Dose
Diphenhydramine	IV: 1 mg/kg (max 50mg)
Hydroxyzine	PO: 0.6 mg/kg/dose q 6 hours (max 50 mg/day)
	IM: 0.5–1 mg/kg/dose q 4–6 hours prn
Metoclopromide	IV: 0.1 mg/kg (max dose 10 mg)
Ondansetron	PO: 4 mg (ages 4–11 years)
	4–8 mg (ages >11 years)
	IV: 0.15 mg/kg/dose (max dose 4 mg)
Prochlorperazine	IV: 0.15 mg/kg (8–17 years) (max dose 10 mg)
Promethazine	IV: 0.5 mg/kg
	IM: 0.5 mg/kg
	PO: 0.25–0.5 mg/kg/dose

Figure 15 Commonly used anti-emetics. *Adverse effects include dystonic reactions and oculogryric crisis (managed with intravenous [IV] benadryl). IM, intramuscular; PO, orally/by mouth; prn, as needed.

Preventive therapies

A diverse group of medications are used to prevent attacks of migraine and it is useful to become comfortable with a few of these agents (Figure 16). Their use should, however, be limited to those patients whose headaches occur with sufficient frequency or severity as to warrant a daily treatment program. Most clinical studies require a minimum of three headaches/month to justify a daily agent. A clear sense of *functional disability* must be established before committing to a course of daily medication. It is also useful to identify the presence of co-morbid conditions (eg depression, obesity) which may suggest the relative benefit of one agent over another.

Once preventive treatment is initiated, patience must be encouraged to permit enough time for the beneficial effects to be appreciated. Generally, an 8–12 week course is necessary before we can determine success or failure. This must be emphasized at the point that the prescriptions are provided, since many impatient families will expect immediate effects after the first days of treatment. We see many patients in our practice who have failed multiple prophylactic courses, only to find the therapeutic trials were only a few days each.

The duration of treatment is controversial. In recognition of the cyclical nature of migraine, the daily agents should be used for a finite period of time. The general recommendation is to provide treatment through the calendar school year, then gradually eliminate daily agents during summer vacation. Another option in younger children is to use a shorter course (eg 6–8 weeks), followed by a slow wean off the medicine.

For preventive or prophylactic treatment in the population of children and adolescents with frequent, disabling migraine, flunarezine, unavailable in the U.S., has established and reproducible efficacy data, but encouraging data is emerging regarding several anti-epileptic agents such as topiramate, divalproex sodium, levateracetam, as well as the antihistamine cyproheptadine and the antidepressant amitriptyline (Figure 16) [89-92].

Options for preventative agents for pediatric migraine

Drug	Dose	Available form	Toxicity
Antihistamines			
Cyproheptadine	0.25–1.5 mg/kg	2 mg/tsp syrup 4 mg tablet	Sedation Weight gain
Anticonvulsants			
Topiramate	1–10 mg/kg/day (usual 50 mg bid)	15, 25 mg sprinkles 25, 100 mg tablets	Sedation Paresthesias Weight loss Glaucoma Kidney stones
Divalproex sodium	20–40 mg/kg/day (usual 250 mg bid)	250 mg/tsp syrup 125 mg sprinkles 250, 500 mg ER tablets	Weight gain Bruising Hair loss Hepatotoxicity Ovarian cysts
Antidepressants			
Amitriptyline	10–50 mg qhs	10, 25, 50 mg tablets	Sedation
Nortriptyline	10–75 mg qhs	10, 25, 50, 75 mg tablets	Weight gain
NSAIDs			
Naproxen sodium	250–500 mg bid	220, 250, 375, 500 mg tablets	Gastritis Nephritis
Calcium channel blockers			
Verapamil	4–10 mg/kg/day tid	40, 80, 120 mg tablets	Hypotension Nausea AV block Weight gain
Beta blockers*			
Propranolol	2–4 mg/kg/day	10, 20, 40, 60, 80 mg tablets 60, 80, 120, 160 mg LA capsules	Hypotension Sleep disorder Decreased stamina Depression

Figure 16 Options for preventative agents for pediatric migraine. *AVOID in patients with asthma, diabetes and depression. ER, extended release; LA, long acting; NSAIDs, non-steroidal anti-inflammatory drugs; SR, sustained release; AV, atrioventricular.

The evidence for preventive treatments in children and adolescents

Antihistamines

Cyproheptadine is an antihistamine with both anti-serotonergic and calcium channel blocker properties which is widely used for migraine prevention in young children (generally age <12 years), but has not been subjected to controlled trials.

For young children, age <10 years without problems of being overweight, cyproheptadine at a starting dose of 2–4 mg as a single bedtime dose is a simple and safe strategy. The doses may be gradually elevated to twice or even three times a day schedules, but, in my experience, most children become too sedated at doses much higher than 4–8 mg/day.

One retrospective study of the use of preventative agents for children and adolescents with migraine within one pediatric neurology practice found that headache frequency was reduced from a mean baseline of 8.4 to 3.7 headaches/month with doses ranging between 2–6 mg given at bedtime or divided twice a day. A positive response rate, defined as an overall favorable decrease in headache frequency and intensity plus acceptability of the agent, was noted in 83% (n=30). Common side effects included sedation and increased appetite [93].

Dosing schedules can vary widely from single bedtime schedules to tid regimens. A dose of 2–4 mg po at bedtime is a rational starting point with option to increase to a maximum of 12–16 mg/day divided three times/day. Doses >8 mg/day often cause excess sedation.

Cyproheptadine has two major limiting features: sedation and appetite stimulation. These effects restrict its acceptability in adolescence, but may be advantageous in thin pre-adolescents.

Antidepressants

Amitriptyline has never been assessed in controlled fashion, but remains one of the most widely used agents. Starting doses of 5–10 mg at bedtime may be gradually increased toward 1 mg/kg/day. Controversy exists whether or not pre-treatment electrocardiogram (ECG) is warranted, but I generally do not order ECGs for children on low doses (10–25 mg).

Antidepressants have become a mainstay of migraine prevention in children and adolescents. Two uncontrolled series have been published for pediatric and adolescent migraine which supports the role of amitriptyline. No blinded trials exist. There is ample data to support the efficacy of antidepressants for adult migraine.

The first pediatric study included series of 192 children with headache, of whom 70% had migraine. The average age was 12 years and the patients had more than three headaches/month. They were treated in an open-label fashion with amitriptyline up to a dose of 1 mg/kg/day. An overall reduction in headache frequency and severity was reported in 84%. Looking specifically at the migraine subset, there was a statistically significant reduction in headache frequency and severity, while the duration of headache attacks was unchanged when compared to initiation of the drug. Side effects were minimal [94].

The second study was a retrospective review of the use of preventative agents for children and adolescents within one child neurology practice found that amitriptyline produced a positive response rate of 89% (n=73). Positive response rate was defined as an overall decrease in headache frequency and intensity plus acceptability of the agent. Headache frequency was reduced from a mean baseline of 11 to 4.1 headaches/month. The principal side effect was mild sedation [93].

The tricyclic antidepressants *amitriptyline*, *nortriptyline*, and *desimpramine* are widely employed and selection is generally a matter of personal preference and experience. There are no comparative data.

Amitriptyline is started as a single bedtime dose of 5–10 mg and slowly, every 4–6 weeks, titrated upward, as necessary, toward 25–50 mg. Sedation is the primary complication. Advantages of amitriptyline include low cost and its once-a-day schedule, which improves compliance. ECG may be warranted if doses in higher ranges (>25–50 mg/day) are used.

The selective serotonin reuptake inhibitors (SSRI) may have a role in those children and adolescents with migraine and co-morbid anxiety, depression, or obsessive-compulsive disorder. No controlled studies have been performed in children or adolescents. A morning dose of 10–20 mg of fluoxetine (Prozac™) may be considered in this population, but caution must be exercised given recent FDA black box warning regarding suicide risks in adolescents with this class of antidepressants. Caution should be exercised when considering use of a triptan in patients taking SSRIs since there is a risk of serotonin toxicity.

Antiepileptic drugs

Topiramate is gaining wide acceptance since mounting evidence, based on well designed controlled trials, support its use. A 26 week trial of 50, 100, and 200 mg doses of topiramate found a reduction in monthly migraine frequency of 46%, 63% and 65% vs 16% with placebo [95]. A second trial evenly randomized 44 children to receive 100 mg divided twice a day vs placebo and found a reduction in the mean monthly migraine attacks was 16/month to 4/month in the treatment group vs 13/month to 8/month (p=0.025) [96]. In this study, there was a significant reduction in overall disability and in school absenteeism. A third, recent report comparing 50mg/day vs 100mg/day versus matched placebo found statistically significant improvement from the prospective baseline period in migraine frequency in the 100mg dose (75% decrease monthly migraine), but not the 50mg (46% decrease) or the placebo group (45%) (p=0.016). The most benefit was appreciated in 100 mg group (50 mg po bid) in which it was observed that over 80% of patients experienced a >50% reduction in headache burden after about eight weeks of treatment [97].

Typically, for teenagers, a dose of 15–25 mg of topiramate is initiated as a single bedtime dose and then gradually titrated toward 50 mg bid incrementally on a weekly or every-other week basis. Clinical experience has demonstrated that many patients will respond with doses as low as 25 mg at bedtime, so it is valuable to titrate to desired effect. Cognitive effects must be monitored quite carefully and more evidence is needed to assess the educational impact of topiramate for prevention of adolescent migraine. It is counterproductive to reduce the headache burden at the expense of academic performance.

Disodium valproate has strong efficacy data in adults and is approved for use as a migraine preventative agent, but no controlled trials exist in children or adults. Several long-term open label trials have demonstrated safety and tolerability [98].

Disodium **valproate** was reported in a retrospective study of for migraine prophylaxis in children, ages 7–16 years (n=42) at a dosing range of 15–45 mg/kg/day which found that 81% were successful in discontinuing all acute medications. After four months of treatment, 75.8% of the patients reported a 50% reduction in headache frequency, 14.2% had a 75% reduction and 14.2% achieved a headache-free status. Side effects included GI upset, weight gain, somnolence, dizziness, and tremor, similar to those experienced by patients with epilepsy [99].

A second study using sodium valproate included children age 9–17 years (n=10) who were treated in an open-label fashion with doses between 500–1000 mg. Both headache severity and frequency were reduced. Mean severity at baseline using a visual analog scale was reduced from 6.8 to 0.7 at the end of treatment (p=0.000). Mean headache attacks/month were reduced from 6/month to 0.7/month and mean duration of headache attack was reduced from 5.5 hours to 1.1 hours following treatment. Side effects included dizziness, drowsiness, and increased appetite, but no serious side effects were noted in this small study. The authors conclude that divalproex sodium is safe and effective for migraine prophylaxis in children [90].

The doses used for valproate are lower than those used for seizure control. A schedule of 10 mg/kg/day or 250 mg po bid or a single bedtime dose of the extended release preparation (250 mg, 500 mg), is a rational starting point. A similar monitoring schedule to that used for patients taking valproate for epilepsy applies with periodic measurements of blood counts, especially platelets, liver chemistries and amylase.

The acceptability of valproate in adolescent females warrants caution in view of the appetite stimulation and risk of ovarian dysfunction (eg polycystic ovary).

Levetiracetam has open label data from 19 patients (mean age 11.9 years) whose mean migraine frequency fell from 6.3 migraine/month to 1.7/month at doses of 125–250 mg bid. Ten patients (52.6%) had complete resolution of headache. The authors concluded that levetiractam appeared to be a promising candidate for well-controlled clinical trials of pediatric patients with migraine [100]. A second open-label trial of 20 patients found that 18/20 patients had ≥50% reduction in monthly migraine frequency and had lowered disability scales at doses of about 20 mg/kg/day [101].

Levetiracetam at doses of 125–250 mg bid was assessed in a retrospective fashion including 19 patients (mean age 12 years) treated for a mean duration of 4.1 months. The average frequency of headache attacks before treatment was 6.3/month and after treatment, fell to 1.7/month (p<0.0001). A striking 52% of patients experienced elimination of migraine attacks during treatment. No side effects were reported in 82.4% but 10.5% discontinued treatment because of side effects including somnolence, dizziness, and irritability. These impressive results suggest a need for controlled trial.

Gabapentin was reported to be effective in one small retrospective study (n=18) in children using doses of 15 mg/kg. Over 80% of patients experienced a more than 50% reduction in headache frequency and severity [102]. Perhaps the most desirable feature of gabapentin is the low incidence of side effects.

Zonisamide was also reported to be effective in one small open label study in children (10–17 years) with mixed, refractory headache conditions (50% migraine). Patients were treated with an average dose of 6 mg/kg/day [103]. Two-thirds had a greater than 50% reduction in headache frequency from baseline.

Anti-hypertensive agents
Beta-blockers
Once widely felt to be the drug of choice for migraine, **propranolol** has been studied in three randomized, double-blind studies, but the results have *failed*

to consistently demonstrate effectiveness. While beta-blockers are still viewed as one of the first line agents in adult migraine, they have a limited role in pediatrics and adolescents.

The first study did show effectiveness and was a double-blind, crossover trial in children age 7–16 years (n=28) using 60–120 mg/day (0.5–1 mg/kg/day divided three times/day). Among the propranolol treated patients, 20/28 patients (71%) had complete remission from headaches and another three patients (10%) experienced a 66% reduction in headache frequency. In the placebo group, 3/28 had complete remission and 1/28 experienced a 66% improvement. The author concluded that propranolol has an "excellent prophylactic effect" for children with frequent and severe attacks of migraine [104].

A second study (n=39) failed to demonstrate benefit using slightly higher doses of 80–120mg/day and, in fact, showed a significant *increase* in the average duration of headache in the propranolol treatment group [105]. A third trial compared propranolol at a dose of 3mg/kg/day vs self-hypnosis and found no benefit from propranolol but significant improvement with hypnotherapy [106]. Propranolol may be used on a single long acting daily dose (LA) form or on a two or three times/day schedule. The LA preparation is most useful. The starting dose is 1–2 mg/kg/day and slowly escalated to 3 mg/kg/day as tolerated. Dosing adjustments can be made every two to three weeks.

Another beta-blocker, **timolol** was assessed in a randomized crossover trial with eight weeks in each arm and a four week washout period between arms (n=19). Headache attacks were reduced from 1.37/week at baseline to 0.23/week in the timolol group. In the placebo group, attacks were reduced from 1.06/week baseline to 0.59/week. The authors reported no significant beneficial effect from timolol [107].

The selective beta-blockers **atenolol**, **metoprolol**, and **nadolol** are alternative choices, but there is no data to suggest any relative advantage of one versus another.

Beta-blockers as a group are contra-indicated in the presence of reactive airway disease, diabetes mellitus, orthostatic hypotension and certain cardiac disorders associated with bradyarrhythmias. Curiously, however, a subset of patients with neurocardiogenic syncope and comorbid migraine do very well with propranolol.

Special caution must be made about the use of beta-blockers in two other populations: athletes and patients with affective disorders, particularly depressions. Athletes may experience a lack of stamina and decreased performance. Those children with co-morbid affective disorders can experience deterioration of mood, even suicidal depression, with propranolol.

Calcium channel blockers

Calcium channel blockers are thought to exert their anti-migraine effects by way of selective inhibition of vasoactive substances on cerebrovascular smooth muscle.

Nimodipine (10–20 mg tid) was studied in a single blind, controlled, crossover trial including children ages 7–18 years (n=37), but the results were inconsistent between the two treatment phases. During the first treatment period, there was no difference between active and placebo. Headache frequency/month fell from 3.3 to 2.8 in the active group and from 3.0 to 2.5 in the placebo group (n=NS). During the second treatment phase, there was a significant reduction in headache frequency in the nimodipine group, but there was no effect on headache duration. Side effects were limited to mild abdominal discomfort in >1% [108].

Flunarizine is a remarkable calcium channel blocker that has been evaluated in several well controlled trials. Two double-blind, placebo-controlled trials using 5 mg bedtime doses of flunarizine (n=105) and demonstrated significant reduction in headache frequency in both studies, one also showing decreased headache duration [109,110]. In this first trial, the number of headaches was reduced from a baseline of 8.66 over three months to 2.95 attacks during treatment. Of patients taking flunarizine, 76% noted a ≥50% improvement, whereas only 19% taking placebo had ≥50% improvement. Another open-label trial of 13 patients showed decreased headache frequency [111]. Other than sedation (9.5%) and weight gain (22.2%), side effects were minimal.

Based upon this strong data, the 2004 AAN Practice Parameter for the treatment of pediatric migraine found (paradoxically) that "flunarizine is *probably effective* for preventive therapy and can be considered for this purpose but it is not available in the United States" [16].

Non-steroidal anti-inflammatory agents

Naproxen sodium has been shown to be effective in adolescent migraine in one small series using a double blind, placebo-controlled crossover design. A reduction in headache frequency was experienced in 60% of the patients and severity with naproxen 250 mg bid, whereas only 40% responded favorably to placebo. The rate limiting effect is GI discomfort (48%) [112] for that reason, use should be limited to no more than 6–8 weeks' duration.

Chapter 4

Status migraine: The emergency department management of status migraine

The formal definition of status migraine is persistence of symptoms for >72 hours. This definition is clinically impractical and any persistent, protracted, and debilitating migraine attack that has been unresponsive or intractable to out-patient measures (ie oral, intranasal, sublingual, or subcutaneous measures) and requires urgent medical intervention with parenteral agents ought to be considered status migraine. These patients often present to EDs or urgent care clinics for care and a systematic approach with a series of option must be available.

The five key elements are hydration, analgesia, specific anti-migraine agents, anti-emetics, and sedation. Figure 17 provides a step-wise series of suggestions.

These patients have often been anorectic or have been vomiting and require hydration. Therefore, IV fluid bolus (10-20 cc/kg) with isotonic solution followed by maintenance plus deficit volumes using glucose containing solutions (D5 ½ NS with KCl) is imperative. Their hydration status should be monitored by urine output and by checking urinalysis and/or serum electrolytes.

For analgesia, there are many options including triptan agents (discussed earlier), or ketorolac. Use of narcotics is discouraged because of the attendant nausea and abuse potential.

The migraine specific regimens include the triptan agents, IV divalproex sodium (Depacon™) and DHE, **not** used together. Subcutaneous sumatriptan at a dose of 0.06 mg/kg (max 6 mg) is particularly useful in patients intolerant of oral medications.

IV divalproex sodium, given as a rapid infusion of about 20 mg/kg or a maximum of 1000 mg, though not studied in any controlled fashion, has been reported to have very favorable results [113].

DHE should be considered for the management of status migraine. DHE should not be used if the patient has taken a triptan agent within the previous

24 hours. Prior to initiating an IV DHE protocol, it is recommended to give an IV antiemetic (eg metoclopromide, ondansetron). Toxicities of DHE are infrequent, but vomiting can occur.

The adult dose is 1 mg IV. In children and adolescents, the dose of DHE should be scaled back to minimize adverse events (vomiting and flushing);

- ages 6–9 years, 0.1 mg/dose;
- ages 9–12 years, 0.2 mg/dose;
- ages 12–16 years, 0.3–0.5 mg/dose [114].

Sedation is often useful, particularly if the first wave of treatment fails to produce any appreciable impact of the headache. Sleep has wonderful beneficial effects. Diphenhydramine, 25–50 mg IV, is often quite effective and, when given with the dopaminergic anti-emetics, lessens any probability of dystonic reactions. Benzodiazepines have sedative and anxiolytic properties, valuable in status migraine

The role of low flow oxygen is controversial. Some centers routinely give patients ½-1 liter/min oxygen, but clinical data to justify this practice is limited.

Many EDs have established clinical pathways for migraine status which have resulted in more efficient care, faster through-put (less time in the ED), and clearer depiction of clinical options (Figure 17).

The emergency department management of status migraine

GENERAL

▲ Weight upon admission:_____kg

▲ Allergies ☐ NKDA Other:_____

▲ V.S. including BP upon admission and then q1 hour x3, then routine.

▲ Pulse oximetry

▲ LOC/neuro/respiratory/hydration/cardiovascular assessment upon admission, then with V.S.

▲ Insert PIV

▲ Assess headache on age appropriate pain scale (FACES)

▲ NS IV bolus_____ml (20 ml/kg) over one hour. Max fluid total of 1 liter.

▲ After NS bolus complete, continue NS at maintenance rate,_____ml/hr. (D5 ½ NS with KCL)

▲ Decrease light in room; minimize noise; limit # visitors; limit/restrict TV/radio

▲ Elevate head of bed to 20-30 degrees.

▲ **Start Oxygen:** ½- 1 liter/min via nasal cannula (optional)

MEDICATION OPTIONS

Anti-emetic:

☐ Prochlorperazine (Compazine®)_____mg IV (8-17 yo = 0.15 mg/kg, max dose 10 mg)

☐ Diphenhydramine (Benadryl®)_____mg IV (1 mg/kg; max dose 50 mg)

☐ Metoclopramide (Reglan®)_____mg IV (0.1 mg/kg; max dose 10 mg)

☐ Ondansetron (Zofran®)_____mg IV (0.15 mg/kg/dose, max dose 4 mg)

First Pain medication (select one):

☐ Ketorolac_____mg IV (0.5 mg/kg; max dose 30 mg)

☐ Sumatriptan_____mg SQ (age >5 yo; ≤20 kg give 3 mg; ≥20 kg give 6 mg)

▲ One hour after pain medication infusion, reassess headache on pain scale

Second line pain medication options:

▲ Attending or Resident to notify Neurology. Then,

☐ Valproate Sodium (Depacon®)_____mg IV (20 mg/kg, up to 1000 mg rapid infusion)

☐ Dihydroergotamine (DHE-45®) 1 mg IV q1 hour x 2 doses (must <u>not</u> have received any form

of a serotonin 5-HT agonist [almotriptan, eletriptan, frovatriptan, naratriptan, rizatriptan,

sumatriptan, tegaserod, zolmitriptan] within the past 24 hours).

☐ magnesium

☐ dexamethasone:

☐ Other medications:

Figure 17 The emergency department management of status migraine. Adapted from Children's Hospital of The King's Daughters designed by Dr Dana Ramirez, Dr Kristin Hutchinson, Dr Donald Lewis.

Chapter 5

Chronic migraine
(aka chronic daily headache)

Many adolescents will report the presence of headache virtually every single day. Chronic, non-progressive, unremitting, daily, or near daily, pattern of headache represents one of the most difficult subsets of headache known as Chronic Daily Headache (CDH). CDH is formally defined as more than four months during which the patient has >15 headaches/month with the headaches last more than four hours/day. The estimated prevalence of CDH in adolescents is approximately 1% and may be as high as 4% of the adult population [115–117]. CDH is very common in referral headache clinics, where up to 15-20% of patients will present with daily or near-daily head pain [118].

Understandably, the quality of life of patients with CDH is significantly influenced and the negative impact extends beyond the affected patient to their family, friends, and society as a whole. The extensive disability that results from CDH can be measured in school absence, abstinence from after-school activities and family discord that invariably results. Therefore early diagnosis and management of frequent or CDH is essential. There are four chronic headache categories;

1. chronic migraine;
2. chronic TTH;
3. new daily persistent headache; and
4. hemicrania continua.

Chronic migraine and chronic TTH usually evolve from episodic migraine or TTH. The new daily persistent headaches appeared to represent a unique entity in which the headache starts quite abruptly without any history of previous headache syndrome, but persists for weeks or months. The family can often remember the exact date that the headache began. Hemicrania continua is uncommon in children with daily or continuous unilateral pain, often around one orbit, with conjunctival injection, lacrimation, rhinorrea, and, occasionally, ptosis. One of the key features of hemicrania continua is responsiveness to indomethacin (25–50 g/day).

Each of these four types of CDH is further separated into those with or without superimposed analgesic overuse. The medications implicated in this analgesic overuse syndrome include most OTC analgesics and decongestants (acetaminophen, aspirin, ibuprofen), opioids, butalbital, isometheptene, benzodiazepines, ergotamine, and triptans [119].

The management of CDH is difficult, but breaking the cycle daily headaches is the principal goal. Pharmacological measures, used in isolation, will be uniformly unsuccessful. It is therefore essential to initiate a multi-disciplined approach with emphasis upon preventive strategies taking precedence over the use of intermittent analgesics. This is a paradigm shift for many families who have focused on intermittent medicines. This population of patients has already likely been overusing OTC analgesic agents, so a fundamental change in treatment philosophy must be taught to the patient and their family.

The first part of this teaching process must be the incorporation of lifestyle changes, such as regulation of sleep and eating habits, regular exercise, identification of triggering factors, stress management biofeedback-assisted relaxation therapy, and bio-behavioral programs psychological or psychiatric intervention.

Lifestyle changes include five major components:

1. Return to the routine of adolescent life (eg regular school attendance).
2. Adequate and regular sleep.
3. Regular exercise (20–30 min/day of aerobic exercise).
4. Balanced nutrition, including avoidance of skipping meals.
5. Adequate oral hydration (5 extra glasses of water/day) with avoidance of caffeine.

There is a growing body of literature demonstrating that many adult women who suffer from frequent or daily headache were victims of sexual abuse as adolescents [120]. This data mandates that practitioners caring for teens with CDH speak privately, compassionately, and confidentially with the patient about any stressors, including being a victim of sexual abuse, which are potential aggravating factors.

The pharmacological treatment of CDH requires an individually tailored regimen with the judicious use of prophylactic and analgesic agents. Recognizing the degree of disability will help guide the aggressiveness of the management.

Preventive therapies used for CDH include tricyclic antidepressants (amitriptyline), antiepileptic agents (eg topiramate, divalproex sodium, gabapentin), beta-blockers (propranolol), calcium channel blockers, and NSAIDs.

When making the choice of drugs, it is important to consider co-morbid conditions. For the patient with difficulty falling asleep, amitriptyline at bedtime may provide dual benefits. Similarly, if there are mild to moderate affective issues, amitriptyline, divalproex sodium, or one of the SSRIs may be beneficial. It there is co-morbid obesity, topiramate may decrease the appetite. Alternatively, if the patient's appetite is low, divalproex sodium often stimulates the appetite. The doses used are shown in Figure 16.

The use of analgesic agents for adolescents with CDH is difficult since most of the children describe continuous or near-continuous pain. When do you give the acute analgesic when the pain is continuous and how do you avoid analgesic overuse? One approach is to graph the pattern of headaches to identify those periods of intense headache, as it stands out from the background pain. At this time, analgesics, including the triptan agents, may be most useful. The key to effective use include of analgesic in the CDH population is to recognize the migraine component of the headache as soon as it starts, using an adequate dose, and avoiding overuse.

The outcome of CDH is poorly understood. One report provides short term follow-up on 24 adolescents, peak age 13 years, with CDH of whom greater than half experienced a >75% reduction in headache frequency and one third a >90% improvement in a six month follow up. A wide variety of preventive agents were employed, but amitriptyline and topiramate provided the largest proportion of successful outcomes.

Chapter 6

Prognosis of childhood migraine

The long term prognosis of adolescents with migraine has not been well studied. Five to seven year follow up studies revealed that 20–25% of adolescents originally diagnosed with migraine have remission of symptoms, 50–60% have persistence of their migraine with aura and 25% converting to TTH. Of those originally with TTH, 20% converted to migraine [121,122]. Monastero et al. evaluated 55 adolescents with migraine who were available for ten year follow up and found that 42% had persistent migraine, 38% had experienced remission, and 20% had transformed to TTH. Interestingly, only migraine without aura persisted through the ten year follow up whereas other migrainous disorders and nonclassifiable headaches did not [123]. The longest follow up available came from Brna et al, with 20 year information on 60 out of an original cohort of 95 from 1983. Of the 60, 27% were headache free, 33% had TTH, 17% had migraine and 23% had both TTH and migraine. Of those with persistent headache, 80% described their headaches as moderate to severe, although an overall improvement was described in 66%. TTH was more likely to remit. Headache severity at diagnosis was the most predictive of headache outcome at 20 years [124]. These data indicate that female gender, migraine severity at diagnosis, and longer duration from time of onset of headache until time of initial medical examination tended toward unfavorable prognosis. Given our current understanding of the long term neuropathological and psychosocial consequences of persistent, frequent migraine, further longitudinal epidemiological study of the evolution of adolescent migraine is imperative.

Conclusions

Migraine is a common, chronic, progressive, and debilitating disorder negatively impacting the lives of millions and the origins of the disability can be traced into childhood and adolescence for the overwhelming majority of adult migraneurs.

There is a wide spectrum of clinical forms, but, in children, the most frequent is *migraine without aura* which is characterized by attacks of frontal or bi-temporal pounding, nauseating headache lasting 1–72 hours. A fascinating and challenging subset known as *migraine with aura* and the periodic syndromes can be associated with frightening focal neurological disturbances and may require careful consideration for the possibility of neoplastic, vascular, metabolic, or toxic disorders.

Migraine treatment philosophy now embraces a balanced approach with both bio-behavioral interventions and pharmacological measures. Treatment decisions must be based upon the disability produced by the headaches, the headache burden. A growing body of controlled pediatric data is beginning to emerge regarding the acute and preventative agents lessening our dependence upon extrapolated adult data.

In the near future, we anticipate further advances in understanding the molecular genetics of migraine, advances which will translate to improved care of the pediatric patient with migraine headache. Furthermore, therapeutic energy expended for our pediatric patients will translate to decreased disability as our patients progress into adulthood, lessening the lifespan burden of migraine.

Pediatricians and other primary care providers stand in a pivotal position to prevent decades of suffering and diminished quality of life directly attributable to migraine by:

- providing accurate diagnosis;
- implementing of lifestyle modifications; and
- aggressive use of pharmacologic measures *during adolescence.*

References

1. Bigal ME, Lipton RB. The prognosis of migraine. Curr Opin Neurol 2008; 21:301–308.
2. Olesen J, Headache Classification Subcommittee. The international classification of headache disorders (ICHD-2). Cephalalgia 2004; 24 (supplement 1):1–151.
3. Rothner AD. The evaluation of Headaches in Children and Adolescents. Semin Pediatr Neurol 1995; 2:109-118.
4. Ferrari A, Spaccapelo L, Gallesi A, Sternieri E. Focus on headache as an adverse reaction to drugs. J Headache Pain 2009; 10:235–239.
5. The Childhood Brain Tumor Consortium. The epidemiology of headache among children with brain tumors. Headache in children with brain tumors. J Neurooncol 1991; 10:31–46.
6. Lewis DW, Ashwal S, Dahl G, et al. Practice parameter: evaluation of children and adolescents with recurrent headaches: report of the Quality Standards Subcommittee of the American Academy of Neurology and the Practice Committee of the Child Neurology Society. Neurology 2002; 59:490–498.
7. Sargent JD, Solbach P. Medical evaluation of migraineurs: review of the value of laboratory and radiologic tests. Headache 1983; 23:62–65.
8. Chen JH, Wang PJ, Young C, et al. Etiological classification of chronic headache in children and their electroencephalographic features. Zhonghua Min Guo Xiao Er Ke Yi Xue Hui Za Zhi 1994; 35:397–406.
9. Kramer U, Nevo Y, Harel S. Electroencephalography in the evaluation of headache patients: a review. Isr J Med Sci 1997; 33:816–820.
10. Whitehouse D, Pappas JA, Escala PH, Livingston S. Electroencephalographic changes in children with migraine. New Engl J Med 1967; 27:23–27.
11. Kinast M, Lueders H, Rothner AD, Erenberg G. Benign focal epileptiform discharges in childhood migraine (BFEDC). Neurology 1982; 32:1309–1311.
12. Ziegler DK, Wong G Jr. Migraine in children: clinical and electroencephalographic study of families: the possible relation to epilepsy. Epilepsia 1967; 8:171–187.
13. Aysun S, Yetük M. Clinical experience on headache in children: analysis of 92 cases. J Child Neurol 1998; 13:202–210.
14. Prensky AL, Sommer D. Diagnosis and treatment of migraine in children. Neurology 1979; 29:506–510.
15. Froelich WA, Carter CC, O'Leary JL, Rosenbaum HE. Headache in childhood. Electroencephalographic evaluation of 500 cases. Neurology 1960; 10:639–642.
16. Practice parameter: the utility of neuroimaging in the evaluation of headache in patients with normal neurologic examinations (summary statement). Report of the Quality Standards Subcommittee of the American Academy of Neurology. Neurology 1994; 44:1353–1354.
17. Maytal J, Bienkowski RS, Patel M, Eviatar L. The value of brain imaging in children with headaches. Pediatrics 1995; 96:413–416.
18. Medina LS, Pinter JD, Zurakowski D et al. Children with headache: clinical predictors of the surgical space-occupying lesions and the role of neuroimaging Radiology 1997; 202:819–824.
19. Dooley JM, Camfield PR, O'Neill M, Vohra A. The value of CT scans for children with headaches. Can J Neurol Sci 1990; 17:309–310.

20. Wöber-Bingöl C, Wöber C, Prayer D, et al. Magnetic resonance imaging for recurrent headache in childhood and adolescence. Headache 1996; 36:83–90.

21. Chu ML, Shinnar S. Headaches in children younger than 7 years of age. Arch Neurol 1992; 49:79–82.

22. Lewis DW, Dorbad D. The utility of neuroimaging in the evaluation of children with migraine or chronic daily headache who have normal neurological examinations. Headache 2000; 40:629–632.

23. Medina LS, Kuntz KM, Pomeroy SL. Children with headache suspected of having a brain tumor: a cost-effectiveness analysis of diagnostic strategies. Pediatrics 2001; 108:255–263.

24. Bille BS. Migraine in school children. A study of the incidence and short-term prognosis, and a clinical, psychological and electroencephalographic comparison between children with migraine and matched controls. Acta Paediatr Suppl 1962; 136:1–151.

25. Deubner DC. An epidemiologic study of migraine and headache in 10-20 year olds. Headache 1977; 17:173–180.

26. Sillanpää M. Changes in the prevalence of migraine and other headache during the first seven school years. Headache 1983; 23:15–19.

27. Dalsgaard-Nielsen T. Some aspects of the epidemiology of migraine in Denmark. Headache 1970; 10:14–23.

28. Stewart WF, Linet MS, Celentano DD, et al. Age and sex-specific incidence rates of migraine with and without visual aura. Am J Epidemiol 1991; 34:1111–1120.

29. Lipton RB, Silberstein SD, Stewart WF. An update on the epidemiology of migraine. Headache 1994; 34:319–328.

30. Mortimer MJ, Kay J, Jaron A. Epidemiology of Headache and Childhood Migraine in an Urban General Practice Using Ad Hoc, Vahlquist and IHS Criteria. Dev Med Child Neuro 1992; 34:1095–1101.

31. Valquist B. Migraine in children. Int Arch Allergy Appl Imunol 1955; 7:348–355.

32. Small P, Waters WE. Headache and migraine in a comprehensive school. In: *The Epidemiology of Migraine*. Edited by Waters. Bracknell-Berkshire, England: Boehringer Ingelhelm, Ltd. 1974.

33. Sillanpää M. Prevalence of migraine and other headache in Finnish children starting school. Headache 1976; 15:288–290.

34. Laurell K, Larsson B, Eeg-Olofsson O. Prevalence of headache in Swedish schoolchildren, with a focus on tension-type headache. Cephalalgia 2004; 24:380–388.

35. Stewart WF, Lipton RB, Celentano DD, Reed ML. Prevalence of migraine headache in the United States. JAMA 1992; 267:64–69.

36. Galletti F, Cupini LM, Corbelli I, et al. Pathophysiological basis for migraine prophylaxis. Prog Neurobiol 2009; 89:176–192.

37. Hachinski VC, Porchawka J, Steele JC. Visual symptoms in the migraine syndrome. Neurology 1973; 23:570–579.

38. Parisi P, Villa MP, Pelliccia A, et al. Panayiotopoulos syndrome: diagnosis and management. Neurol Sci 2007; 28:72–79.

39. Kirchmann M, Thomsen LL, Olesen J. Basilar-type migraine; clinical, epidemiologic, and genetic features. Neurololgy 2006; 66:880–886.

40. DeFusco M, Marconi R, Silvestri L, et al. Haploinsufficiency of ATP1A2 encoding Na+/K+ pump alpha-2 subunit associated familial hemiplegic migraine, type 2. Nat Genet 2003; 33:192–196.

41. Dichgans M, Freilinger T, Eckstein G, et al. Mutation in the neuronal voltage-gated sodium channel SCN1A in familial hemiplegic migraine. Lancet 2005; 366:371–377.

42. Cuvellier JC, Lépine A. Childhood periodic syndromes.Pediatr Neurol 2010; 42:1–11.

43. Giffin NJ, Benton S, Goadsby PJ. Benign paroxysmal torticollis of infancy: four new cases and linkage to CACNA1A mutation. Dev Med Child Neurol. 2002; 44:490–493.

44. Silberstein SD. Practice parameter: evidence-based guidelines for migraine headache (an evidence-based review): report of the Quality Standards Subcommittee of the American Academy of Neurology. Neurology 2000; 55:754–762.

45. Powers SW, Patton SR, Hommel KA, Hershey AD. Quality of life in childhood migraine: clinical impact and comparison to other chronic illnesses. Pediatrics 2003; 112:e1–5.

46. Powers SW, Patton SR, Hommell, KA, Hershey AD. Quality of life in paediatric migraine: characterization of age-related effects using PedsQL 4.0. Cephalalgia 2004; 24:120–127.

47. Miller VA, Palermao TM, Powers SW, et al. Migraine Headaches and sleep distrurbances in children. Headache 2003; 43:362–368.

48. Köseoglu E, Akboyraz A, Soyuer A, Ersoy AO. Aerobic exercise and plasma beta endorphin levels in patients with migrainous headache without aura. Cephalalgia. 20030; 23:972–976.

49. Millichap JG, Yee MM. The diet factor in pediatric and adolescent migraine. Pediatr Neurol 2003; 28:9–15.

50. Stang PE, Yanagihara PA, Swanson JW, et al. Incidence of migraine headache: a population based study in Olmsted Country, Minnesota. Neurology 1992; 42:1657–1662.

51. Van den Bergh V, Amery WK, Waelkens J. Trigger factors in migraine: a study conducted by the Belgian Migraine Society. Headache 1987; 27:191–196.

52. James JE. Acute and chronic effects of caffeine on performance, mood, headache, and sleep. Neuropsychobiology 1998; 38:32–41.

53. Mannix LK, Frame JR, Soloman GD. Alcohol, smoking and caffeine use among headache patients. Headache 1997; 37:572–576.

54. Van Dusseldorp M, Katan M. Headache caused by caffeine withdrawal among moderate caffe drinkers switched from ordinary to decaffeinated coffee: a 12 week double-blind trial. BMJ 1990; 300:1558–1559.

55. Trautmann E, Lackschewitz H, Kröner-Herwig B. Psychological treatment of recurrent headache in children and adolescents--a meta-analysis. Cephalalgia. 2006; 26:1411–1426.

56. Zeltzer LK, Schlank CB. *Conquering Your Child's Chronic Pain: A Pediatrician's Guide for Reclaiming a Normal Childhood, 1st Edition*. New York, USA: Harper Paperbacks, 2005.

57. Schürks M, Diener HC, Goadsby P. Update on the prophylaxis of migraine. Curr Treat Options Neurol 2008; 10:20–29.

58. Oelkers-Ax R, Leins A, Parzer P, et al. Butterbur root extract and music therapy in the prevention of childhood migraine: an explorative study. European J Pain 2008; 12:301–313.

59. Hershey AD, Powers SW, Vockell AL, et al. Coenzyme Q10 deficiency and response to supplementation in pediatric and adolescent migraine. Headache 2007; 47:73–80.

60. Lewis D, Ashwal S, Hershey A, et al. Practice parameter: pharmacological treatment of migraine headache in children and adolescents: report of the American Academy of Neurology Quality Standards Subcommittee and the Practice Committee of the Child Neurology Society. Neurology 2004; 63:2215–2224.

61. Victor S, Ryan S. Drugs for preventing migraine headaches in children. Cochrane Database Syst Rev 2003; 4:CD002761.

62. Lewis DW, Yonker M, Winner P, Sowell M. The treatment of pediatric migraine. Pediatr Ann 2005; 34:448–460.

63. Hämäläinen ML. Migraine in children and adolescents; a guide to drug treatment. CNS Drugs 2006; 20:813–820.

64. Gunner KB, Smith HD, Ferguson LE. Practice guideline for the diagnosis and management of migraine headaches in children and adolescents: part two. J Pediatr Health Care; 2008; 22:52–59.

65. Reimschisel T. Breaking the cycle of medication overuse headache. Contemporary Pediatrics 2003; 20:101.

66. Rothner A, Guo Y. An analysis of headache types, over-the-counter (OTC) medication overuse and school absences in a pediatric/adolescent headache clinic. Headache 2004; 44:490.

67. Major PW, Grubisa HS, Thie NM. Triptans for the treatment of acute peditric migraine: a systematic literature review. Pediatr Neurol 2003; 29:425–429.

68. Silver S, Gano D, Gerretsen P. Acute treatment of paediatric migraine; a meta-analysis of efficacy. J Paediatr Child Health 2008; 44:3–9.

69. Hämäläinen ML, Hoppu K, Valkeila E, Santavuori P. Ibuprofen or acetaminophen for the acute treatment of migraine in children: a double-blind, randomized, placebo-controlled, crossover study. Neurology 1997; 48:103–107.

70. Lewis DW, Kellstein D, Dahl G, et al. Children's Ibuprofen Suspension for the Acute Treatment of Pediatric Migraine Headache. Headache. 2002; 42:780–786.

71. Winner P, Rothner AD, Saper J, et al. A randomized, double-blind, placebo-controlled study of sumatriptan nasal spray in the treatment of acute migraine in adolescents. Pediatrics 2000; 106:989–997.

72. Ahonen K, Hämäläinen ML, Rantala H, Hoppu K. Nasal sumatriptan is effective in the treatment of migraine attacks in children Neurology 2004; 62:883–887.

73. Ueberall M. Sumatriptan in paediatric and adolescent migraine. Cephalalgia 2001; 21 (Suppl 1):21–24.

74. Lewis DW, Winner P, Hershey AD, Wasiewski WW. Adolescent Migraine Steering Committee. Efficacy of zolmitriptan nasal spray in adolescent migraine. Pediatrics. 2007; 120:390–396

75. Ahonen K, Hämäläinen ML, Eerola M, Hoppu K. A randomized trial of rizatriptan in migraine attacks in children. Neurology. 2006; 67:1135–1140.

76. Linder SL, Mathew NT, Cady RK, et al. Efficacy and tolerability of Almotriptan in Adolescents; A randomized, double-blind, placebo-controlled trial. Headache 2008; 48:1326–1336.

77. Brandes JL, Kudrow D, Stark SR, et al. Sumatriptan-naproxen for acute treatment of migraine: a randomized trial. JAMA 2007; 297:1443–1454.

78. Haberer LJ, Walls CM, Lener SE, et al. Distinct pharmacokinetic profile and safety of a fixed-dose tablet of sumatriptan and naproxen sodium for the acute treatment of migraine. Headache 2010; 50:357–373.

79. Evers S, Rahmann A, Kraemer C, et al. Treatment of childhood migraine attacks with oral zolmitriptan and ibuprofen. Neurology. 2006; 67:497–499.

80. McEnroe JD, Fleishaker JC. Clinical pharmacokinetics of almotriptan, a serotonin 5-HT1B/1D receptor agonist for the treatment of migraine. Clin Pharmacokinet 2005; 44:237–246.

81. Charles JA. Almotriptan in the acute treatment of migraine in patients 11-17 years old: an open-label pilot study of efficacy and safety. Headache Pain 2006; 7:95–7.

82. Berenson F, Vasconcellos E, Pakalnis A, et al. Long-term, open-label safety study of oral almotriptan 12.5 mg for the acute treatment of migraine in adolescents. Headache 2010;50(5):795-807.

83. Winner P, Lewis D, Visser WH, et al. Rizatriptan 5 mg for the acute treatment of migraine in adolescents: a randomized, double-blind placebo-controlled study. Headache 2002; 42:49–55.

84. Winner P, Pensky A, Linder S. Efficacy and safety of oral sumatriptan in adolescent migraines. Presented at: *American Association for the Study of Headache* meeting; Chicago. May 1996.

85. Ueberall MA. Intranasal sumatriptan for the acute treatment of migraine in children. Neurology 1999; 52:1507–1510.

86. Linder SL. Subcutaneous sumatriptan in the clinical setting: the first 50 consecutive patients with acute migraine in a pediatric neurology office practice. Headache 1996; 36:419–422.

87. Linder SL, Dowson AJ. Zolmitriptan provides effective migraine relief in adolescents. Int J Clin Pract 2000; 54:466–469.

88. Lewis DW, Winner P, Hershey AD, Wasiewski WW. Efficacy of zolmitriptan nasal spray in adolescent migraine. Pediatrics 2007; 120:390–396.

89. Hershey AD, Powers SW, Vockell AL, et al. Effectiveness of topiramate in the prevention of childhood headache. Headache 2002; 42:810–818.

90. Serdaroglu G, Erhan E, Tekgul, et al. Sodium valproate prophylaxis in childhood migraine. Headache 2002; 42:819–822.

91. Eiland LS, Jenkins LS, Durham SH. Pediatric migraine; pharmacologic agents for prophylaxis. Ann Pharmacother 2007; 41:1181–1190.

92. Damen L, Bruijn J, Verhagen AP, et al. Prophylactic treatment of migraine in children. A systematic review of pharmacological trials. Cephalalgia 2006; 26:497–505.

93. Lewis DW, Diamond S, Scott D, Jones V. Prophylactic treatment of pediatric migraine. Headache 2004; 44:230–237.

94. Hershey AD, Powers SW, Bentti AL, Degrauw TJ. Effectiveness of amitriptyline in the prophylactic management of childhood headaches. Headache 2000; 40:539–549.

95. Winner P, Gendolla A, Stayer C, et al. Topiramate for migraine prevention in adolescents: a pooled analysis of efficacy and safety. Headache 2006; 46:1503–1510.

96. Lakshmi CV, Singhi P, Malhi P, Ray M. Topiramate in the prophylaxis of pediatric migraine; a double-blind placebo-controlled trial. J Child Neurol 2007; 22:829–835.

97. Lewis D, Winner P, Saper J, et al. Randomized, double-blind, placebo-controlled study to evaluate the efficacy and safety of topiramate for migraine prevention in pediatric subjects 12 to 17 years of age. Pediatrics. 2009; 123:924–934.

98. Apostol G, Lewis DW, Laforet GA, et al. Divalproex sodium extended-release for the prophylaxis of migraine headache in adolescents: results of a stand-alone, long-term open-label safety study. Headache 2009; 49:45–53.

99. Caruso JM, Brown WD, Exil G, Gascon GG. The efficacy of divalproex sodium in the prophylactic treatment of children with migraine. Headache 2000; 40:672–676.

100. Miller GS. Efficacy and safety of levetiracetam in pediatric migraine. Headache 2004; 44:238–243.

101. Pakalnis A, Kring D, Meier L. Levetiracetam prophlyaxis in pediatric migraine – an open label study. Headache 2007; 47:427–430.

102. Belman AL, Milazo M, Savatic M. Gabapentin for Migraine Prophylaxis in Children. Annals of Neurology 2001; 50 (Suppl 1):S109.

103. Pakalnis A, Kring D. Zonisamide prophylaxis in refractory pediatric headache. Headache 2006; 46:804–807.

104. Ludvigsson J. Propranolol used in prophylaxis of migraine in children. Acta Neurol Scand 1974; 50:109–115.

105. Forsythe WI, Gillies D, Sills MA. Propranolol ('Inderal') in the treatment of childhood migraine. Dev Med Child Neuro1984; 26:737–741.

106. Olness K, MacDonald JT, Uden DL. Comparison of Self-Hypnosis and Propranolol in the Treatment of Juvenile Classic Migraine. Pediatrics 1987; 79:593–597.

107. Noronha MJ. Double-blind randomized cross-over trial of timolol in migraine prophylaxis in children. Cephalalgia 1985; 5 (Suppl 3):174–175.

108. Battistella PA, Ruffilli R, Moro R, et al. A placebo-controlled crossover trial of nimodipine in pediatric migraine. Headache 1990; 30:264–268.

109. Sorge F, Marano E. Flunarizine V. placebo in childhood migraine. A double-blind study. Cephalalgia 1985; 5 (Suppl 2):145–148.

110. Sorge F, DeSimone R, Marano E, et al. Flunarizine in prophylaxis of childhood migraine. A double-blind, placebo-controlled crossover study. Cephalalgia 1988; 8:1–6.

111. Guidetti V, Moscato D, Ottaviano S, et al. Flunarizine and migraine in childhood an evaluation of endocrine function. Cephalalgia 1987; 7:263–266.

112. Lewis DW, Middlebrook MT, Deline C. Naproxen Sodium for Chemoprophylaxis of Adolescent Migraine. Ann Neurol 36; 542:1994.

113. Norton J. Use of intravenous valproate sodium in status migraine. Headache 2000; 40:755–757.

114. Linder SL. Treatment of childhood headache with dihydroergotamine mesylate. Headache. 1994; 34:578–580.

115. Abu-Arefeh I, Russell G. Prevalence of headache and migraine in schoolchildren. BMJ 1994; 309:765–769.

116. Lipton R, Stewart W. Prevalence and impact of migraine. Neurol. Clin 1997; 15:1–13.

117. Castillo J, Muñoz P, Guitera V, Pascual J. Kaplan Award 1998. Epidemiology of chronic daily headache in the general population. Headache 1999; 39:190–196.

118. Viswanathan V, Bridges SJ, Whitehouse W, Newton RW. Childhood headaches: discrete entities or continuum? Dev Med Child Neurol. 1998; 40:544–550.

119. Mathew NT, Kurman R, Perez F. Drug-induced refractory headache- clinical features and management. Headache 1990; 30:634–638.

120. Tietjen GE, Brandes JL, Digre KB, et al. History of childhood maltreatment is associated with co-morbid depression in women with migraine. Neurology 2007; 69:959–968.

121. Camarda R, Monastero R, Santangela G, et al. Migraine headaches in adolescents: a five year follow up study. Headache 2002; 42:1000–1005.

122. Kienbacher C, Wöber C, Zesch HE, et al. Clinical features, classification and prognosis of migraine and tension-type headache in children and adolescents: a long term follow up study. Cephalalgia 2006; 26:820–830.

123. Monastero R, Camarda C, Pipia C, Camarda R. Prognosis of migraine headaches in adolescents; a 10 year follow-up study. Neurology 2006; 67:1353–1356.

124. Brna P, Dooley J, Gordon K, Dewan T. The prognosis of childhood headache; a 20 year follow up. Arch Pediatr Adolesc Med 2005; 159:1157–1160.